La Leche League

. . . .

La Leche League

At the Crossroads of

Medicine, Feminism,

and Religion

Jule DeJager Ward

The University of
North Carolina Press

Chapel Hill & London

Designed by April Leidig-Higgins
Set in Carter and Cone Galliard
by Keystone Typesetting, Inc.
Manufactured in the United States of America

The paper in this book meets the guidelines for
permanence and durability of the Committee on
Production Guidelines for Book Longevity of the
Council on Library Resources.

Library of Congress Cataloging-in-Publication Data
Ward, Jule DeJager.
La Leche League: at the crossroads of medicine,
feminism, and religion / Jule DeJager Ward.
p. cm. Includes bibliographical references and index.
ISBN 0-8078-2509-3 (cloth: alk. paper).
ISBN 0-8078-4791-7 (pbk.: alk. paper)
1. Breast feeding — Social aspects.
2. Breast feeding — Religious aspects.
I. La Leche League International. II. Title.
RJ216.W37 2000   649'.33 — dc21   99-12921 CIP

04 03 02 01 00   5 4 3 2 1

contents

· ·

illustrations

· ·

preface

· ·

In 1971 I was the mother of a two-year-old daughter and a five-month-old baby girl who had chosen to remain full time with her children rather than return to outside employment. As it had been with both excitement and trepidation that I had given up my position as an assistant editor for a magazine, I was pleasantly surprised to find I was neither isolated nor bored. Career opportunities for women in the late 1960s, however, were not what they would become. At the magazine I had definitely been a second-tier member of the editorial staff with little hope of becoming anything else. At home, my girls presented me with an enjoyable challenge doing important work — although at a rather hectic pace. I had many friends in the community who had also left employment to raise families. We shared recipes, war stories, techniques, and child care.

There was, however, one important area in which I felt distanced from these other women. I was the only one I knew who was breast-feeding her baby. This awareness was particularly acute in the area of sharing child care. Whereas my friends could leave bottles with me for their little ones, I was hampered because my girls hated bottles and refused to take them. Yet, I believed in the "wisdom" of the time that said for my sake and that of my husband I "needed" to leave the baby sometimes. I was in a quandary.

Adding to my confusion, my doctor insisted that my infant was thriving on breast milk and did not need solids. I was certain he was right, but

I found it hard to fend off increasing demands by relatives that I "feed that baby some real food." Then I read an announcement of a La Leche League meeting that would take place three blocks from my house later that week. I decided to attend. That night I felt I had come home at last.

During the years from 1970 to 1983, my involvement with the League grew. First, I became group secretary. Then, I became a leader, leading meetings and counseling mothers with breast-feeding problems. I helped organize the twenty-fifth-anniversary convention in 1981. I wrote for the newsletter and spoke at national and state conferences. I had become a true believer. The League and my family absorbed my life.

In 1983 a new wind swept through my life. Because my fourth and youngest child was starting to attend a full-day school program, I decided to go back to school myself. I resigned from the League. There just was not enough time for three priority commitments, and I was beginning to outgrow the League. Once in school, I discovered that the world of women had changed enormously during my self-imposed isolation from mainstream culture. I began to see feminism in a new light, and because I was pursuing a doctorate in theology, this light was feminist theology.

I also learned to see my faith community, the Roman Catholic Church, through new eyes. I became intrigued by its recent evolution and struggle with the newly emerging roles for women in society. In my first years in graduate school, I never even considered that La Leche League might be part of these concepts. This revelation came when I realized that the League had much in common with the persuasive therapies, ancient, modern, and contemporary. When I put this together with an understanding that all therapy is informed in some way by a religious dimension, I began to ask, What is the religious dimension of La Leche League, how does it function, and what could I learn from exploring this subject? Gradually, this inquiry led to this book.

Seeming to have left the League more than a dozen years ago, I found myself coming back to an almost full-time interest in this organization, but no longer as a "true believer." And yet, I am not a scoffing skeptic either. In fact, my examination of the League renewed my confidence in many of its basic concepts even as this inquiry revealed a certain rigidity in its interpretation of these concepts. No institution that is unwilling to be critically self-reflective can maintain a high standard of service and care. So I offer this descriptive historical critique as a gift to La Leche

League, even though I write now as one removed in time and distance. And, though I strive to maintain an objective distance as I write, I know that this is never completely possible and I am content that it is not. I think too highly of the work of La Leche League to ever want to be completely distanced from it.

This book is dedicated first to all the members of La Leche League, past and present, without whom this narrative could not exist. Second, I dedicate it to my husband, John, for his tireless support as my most enthusiastic copy editor, and to my children — to Carrie and Betsy for believing in me and to Johnny and Kristy for keeping me real. Thanks are also in order for my writing group, Ian Evison, Don Kispert, Barbara McGinnis-Gillespie, and Kathleen Dolphin. The camaraderie of those who struggle together can never be underestimated. The members of my dissertation committee also offered continuing guidance. Don Browning inspired me to see La Leche League as a topic ripe for theological exploration. Martin Marty kept my sense of narrative fresh. Anne Carr's warmth and intelligence directed my exploration of feminism. My thanks go as well to Elaine Maisner, my editor, who was always there with "tea and sympathy" as well as clear and thoughtful direction. To all these people and to those friends who listened and queried through all the ups and downs of writing, I extend my sincere gratitude.

La Leche League

. . . .

introduction

. . . .

La Leche League

Religious Metaphors in a Secular Ethos

This book will present an exploration of a quasi-religious narrative and a history of the impact it has had on millions of individuals within many contemporary cultures. This narrative includes foundational myths, sacred legends, explanatory stories, and moral illustrations that challenge the mind and heart to think and feel differently. Within this narrative, distinctions between what is literal and what is metaphorical blur. Verifiable scientific realities are sometimes unconsciously linked to the metaphors and symbols of Christianity. Thus, it is important to discover how these metaphors and symbols are used in their original sources, because those meanings will color the narrative in unexpected, and perhaps unwanted, ways.

This narrative is the story of La Leche League, an organization founded in 1956 by a group of Catholic mothers who sought to mediate in a comprehensive way between the family and the world of modern technological medicine. From its inception, the League's founders have believed, "[The League] carries with it the hope of rescuing us from a sick technological age by the restoration of certain basic human relations leading to a more wholesome culture."[1]

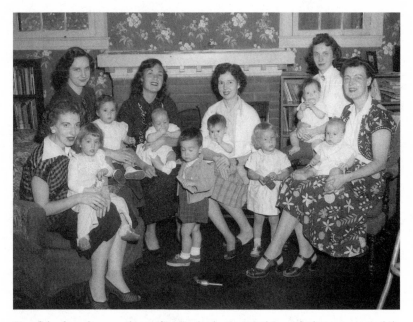

Six of the founding mothers of La Leche League gather with their younger children in 1957. From left to right: Mary Ann Cahill with Mary; Betty Wagner
with Peggy; Mary Ann Kerwin with Tommy and baby Eddie; Mary White with
Michael; Marian Tompson with Laurel and Sheila; and Edwina Froehlich with
Peter. Viola Lennon was not present.

My aim is to enlarge human discourse by revealing the world of La
Leche League as a culture, that is, a context within which behaviors and
processes can be intelligibly described. In order to dissolve the obscurity
of the group's views, this book presents the League to those outside the
group by inviting them within the framework of the League's perceptions. It demonstrates the League's normalness without reducing its
uniqueness. It describes the League's expressed self-perception while in-
terpreting that perception as standing within a broader cultural context.
Here, the emphasis is on exploration and portrayal. The reader enters a
conversation with La Leche League. The goal of the conversation is to
question, listen faithfully, and hear the questions the League asks us. I
have limited negative criticism in order to focus on presenting as clear a
picture as possible of La Leche League. The focus here is the way League
ideology incorporated strands of several late-twentieth-century perspectives. League attitudes and approaches often left out other, perhaps
equally important strands of these same viewpoints. Without neglecting

this fact, this work explores what La Leche League did, not what it failed to do.

This exploration places the League narrative within the various traditions that contributed all unknowingly their wisdom to the philosophy League members call "LLLove." An examination of each of these traditions—the scientific community, the American Catholic Church, and the first stirring of "second-wave" feminism—leads the way to comprehending La Leche League. The League has received some scrutiny from the social sciences. Such approaches are, however, limited and fail to examine the rich diversity of La Leche League's practical wisdom. Understanding the various dimensions of League wisdom also requires examining how they interact with one another. Metaphors from both Catholicism and feminism enliven and give coherence to its basic scientific models.[2]

Finding a way to bring more adequate information to mothers wanting to breast-feed was the impetus that brought together the founders of La Leche League. Relating how they came together and expanded outward begins our story. The ordinariness of their beginnings and the rather typical way they approached their challenge makes the story of their extraordinary success all the more astonishing. But when one looks at the powerful currents of thought that the earliest members both consciously and unconsciously incorporated into their basic ideology, the phenomenal growth of this organization becomes easier to understand. The reality that some aspects of their approach arise from elements in our culture that are open to serious challenge does not render the approach less effective. Indeed, by utilizing, with varying degrees of awareness, tenets already embedded in their culture, League members developed a perspective with established appeal. New scientific technologies, the women's movement, and a strong concern about family life are powerful forces in contemporary society, and all contribute to the League's ideology.

From the perspective of La Leche League's founders, it was the solidity of their scientific knowledge base that grounded the other elements of their philosophy. Although their manual was not intended as a substitute for valuable medical research, they realized that many mothers who wished to breast-feed did not achieve that wish because they had received poor information from the medical community. At the same time, however, they also recognized that good professional help did exist, even if it was rare. La Leche League entered into the dialogue between mothers and medicine midstream. By the middle of the twentieth century the medical profession had taken control of mothering. Most new mothers felt dependent on "experts" to know how to mother. Women's ancient wisdom had been replaced. The League did not seek to replace good scientific information or the proper role of the doctor. Its goal was to help mothers learn to breast-feed by making the best information about breast feeding available to them. League women saw the source of that information as twofold: good medical advice and the experience of mothers who had breast-fed their infants.

A central component of League ideology is that mothers are best suited to help other women learn the arts of mothering. Members exhibit a strong confidence in their ability to effect important changes in their society through woman-to-woman networks. These networks also support League members against the buffetings of the outside world. In these ways their attitudes and actions indicate a feminist bent. However, their beliefs come into conflict with some feminist theories about the mother-child relationship. The relationship between feminism and motherhood is multidimensional. La Leche League's perspective on the family falls within the spectrum of feminist understandings. The League's understanding of feminism and the feminist perspective toward the League, however, have sometimes been characterized most strongly by mutual suspicion. This fact is explored here, but in this work it is neither possible to fully examine the feminist critique of the patriarchal family nor feasible to mount a full-fledged feminist critique of La Leche League. Instead, as the book unfolds, I point out those places where League understandings of women's roles are problematic while I concentrate on the League's promotion of a strong role for women. This stance is surprising in an organization usually associated with a strong traditionalism.

Another central characteristic of La Leche League's ideology is that it was born of Catholic moral discourse on family life and nurtured by the scientific convictions of a sociobiological ethic. The League has very strong convictions about the needs of families. These convictions are the normative heart of its narrative. Personal accounts ring with the intrigue of moral tales. Babies' lives are saved. Disrupted homes are peaceful again. Confused women find a potent meaning to their lives. The League's presentations and literature carry a strong suggestion that breast feeding is obligatory. Their message is simple: Nature intended mothers to nurse their babies; therefore, mothers ought to nurse. This confidence that the nutritional health of the baby and the mother depend on breast feeding is coupled with an equally persuasive belief that the mother's presence is vital to the baby's psychological development.

These beliefs engender two questions. First, does La Leche League's desire to be a free mover in a pluralist society cause it to neglect strengths available in the religious aspects of its ethos? For instance, when League literature depends solely on scientific findings to support its claims, such statements are vulnerable to scientific counterclaims. Conversely, an argument for considering the baby's needs before those of other family members may actually stand on firm moral ground that the League neglects to claim.

An equally important question is whether adherence to unacknowledged religious metaphors for family life weakens the organization's ability to help and counsel contemporary mothers. For instance, the League's uncomplicated assimilation of certain tenets such as male-female complementarity is grounded in traditional Christian beliefs about essential differences between men and women. Many feminists, however, including many Christian writers, question such assumptions. The challenge to this aspect of League ideology often blossoms unnecessarily into an overall critique of the League itself. I myself question both the Catholic and the La Leche League stand on male-female complementarity, but the task here is to compare League understandings on the husband-wife relationship with those of the Catholic Church and to ask what are the strengths and weaknesses of each.

To examine questions such as the last one, it is necessary to include within this story another narrative. This is the history of the American Catholic Church's family theology in the mid-twentieth century. The League founders made a conscious decision to engage in an ongoing conversation with scientific research and to keep their organization pluralist in constituency and secular in ethos. Nevertheless, League philosophy continues to manifest its unconscious religious origins and contains within its practical discourse strands of Catholic social thought on the family. Because Catholic religiosity encompasses beliefs from the various cultures within which it finds expression, certain subtexts of Catholic belief can also be found in La Leche League concepts.

Catholicism encompasses a complex and often confusing understanding of women: it perceives them as subordinate to men in human relationships yet equal with men before God. This tradition often expresses a deep confidence in women's power to effect sweeping community-wide changes yet limits the spheres of that influence. From Catholicism, the League has inherited a strong, structured family value system but also an uncompromising approach to family dynamics. The former assists League members in their work; the latter restricts them by putting them at odds with many contemporary mothers. In this book, the League's positive inheritances from Catholicism, faith in the goodness of family and confidence in women's effectiveness, are emphasized. This emphasis is chosen not because the negative legacy is unimportant but because the simple existence of a parallel between Catholic thought and League ideals is at the heart of this story. It not only colors League understandings of women's roles but transforms their use of scientific findings into a particular perception of the good.

From La Leche League's founding, its roots in Catholicism were denied, ignored, or went unrecognized. Yet, as I illustrate in Chapter 7, League language is steeped in a particular understanding of natural law theory. The ethic of family life finds direct parallels in papal encyclicals. The idealization of motherhood reflects the place of Mary in Catholic popular devotion. And the approach to community strongly resembles that of the Christian Family Movement.

The language of La Leche League is a subtle blend of three different languages: scientific, feminist, and quasi-religious expressions and concepts come together to speak in one voice. This voice expresses the memories, the tradition, and the wisdom of La Leche League today, but like all languages it must either adapt and change or become archaic. If La Leche League is to remain a force for positive change in the world of child care, it must change, and there are strong indications that the League is evolving. It is, however, evolving in its own way. The manner in which League mothers make choices about motherhood duplicates neither the approach of strict traditionalists nor that of liberal feminists. They are forging a singular path, one that can appeal to a broad spectrum of mothers both in the United States and across the world. Its uniqueness assures us that the League will continue to play a positive role in the "politics of the family" in which the world is now engaged. It is just as true that many mothers will find League policies unappealing. This invalidates neither their views nor those of League mothers. It simply means that the La Leche League ideology is one of many good approaches to parenting.

chapter 1

. . . .

What Is La Leche League?

ON A MISSION

Within the field of infant nutrition, the name La Leche League is well known. Parents and those who support them in their parenting endeavors have studied and debated the League's purposes and the way it pursues its goals since its inception in 1956. In spite of its familiarity to parents of babies, the League remains relatively unknown outside this sphere.

La Leche League is a nonprofit, nonsectarian organization dedicated to helping mothers who wish to breast-feed their babies.[1] The League carries out its purpose by holding regular small-group discussions with mothers interested in breast feeding. These discussions take place in a series of meetings led by mothers experienced in breast feeding. These women find satisfaction in helping other mothers breast-feed their infants successfully.[2]

From the League's earliest days, its leaders were able to say with confidence that most doctors agreed that "breast-fed is best fed," and they have always employed the services of a board of medical consultants. These mothers, however, have not believed that doctors are necessarily the best source of direct information for a mother who is considering breast feeding. For League members, the medical community sometimes represented the "hostile technologic culture, prone to scientism and insensitive to and rejective of nature's obvious script."[3] From its inception, La Leche League believed that many questions about nursing a baby could best be answered by experienced mothers. This simple concept became the basis for a global organization.

No one was more surprised by this than the League's seven founding mothers. Dr. Herbert Ratner, the editor of *Child and Family* and a consultant to La Leche League from its inception, noted in 1958, "The momentousness of the birth was only to be appreciated many years later with the development of the modest newborn into a robust, worldwide organization of great influence, whose universal message transcends peoples, nations and governments."[4] How did such growth happen? For one of the founders, Edwina Froehlich, the strength of belief in the importance of their message was what made the League work.

It was as simple as that. This very simplicity gives the story of La Leche League's beginnings an aura of the mythical. On a hot and sunny day in July 1956, two young mothers attended a Christian Family Movement (CFM, earlier known as the Catholic Family Movement) picnic together. Mary White, a doctor's wife, who had breast-fed all but the first of her six children, and her close friend Marian Tompson, who was successfully nursing her fourth child but first breast-fed baby, fed their babies while relaxing under a tree. They shared with one another how fortunate they were to be enjoying the ease and convenience of nursing. Around them other mothers struggled first to keep formula cold enough to remain fresh and then to discover some way to heat it up so that their babies could drink it safely and comfortably. As mother after mother walked over to them and said, "I had so wanted to nurse my baby but . . . ," they began to realized that the difficulties they had encountered in their first attempts at nursing were not rare but were shared by many women. In that moment, they committed themselves to helping community friends who wanted to nurse their babies. They asked each other what had made the difference for them. Both realized it had been the confidence of White's husband, Dr. Gregory White, in their ability to nurse and his assurance that their babies were thriving.

Such assurance was by no means the universal experience of new mothers. Although physicians might lavish praise on breast feeding, at the same time they warned of the difficulties that faced the nursing mother and tended to assume that the mother would end up bottle feeding. Many doctors held that successful breast feeding demanded a knowledge of scientific and medical discoveries. They expected that few mothers would have sufficient quantities of milk to nourish their children. Most mothers were told to make up for this expected "deficiency" by nursing on a strict schedule and by supplementing each feeding with formula.[5]

The founders had no special expertise in teaching women the art of breast feeding. Becoming world leaders in the field of infant nutrition began when they shared their personal stories with other mothers.

White's mother's decision to bottle-feed was influenced by the work of Dr. Emmet Holt, a physician who focused on rigid scheduling in all aspects of infant care, including feeding the baby bottles "by the clock." But White was convinced that formula feeding was no panacea. For one thing, she knew that many formula-fed infants suffered from severe allergies to the ingredients in many artificial formulas. These infants could become very ill before an adequate breast-milk substitute was found. Several of her siblings had suffered from such allergies. Therefore, she had been determined to breast-feed. When her first child was born, however, White followed her mother's advice and supplemented breast feeding with a bottle because she had been told at the hospital that she did not have enough milk. Her baby soon became a completely bottle-fed baby.

Marian Tompson's experiences had been similarly frustrating. Tompson does not recall a specific decision to breast-feed her infants. She assumed that she would breast-feed because she was orientated to the natural. Her faith in breast feeding asserted itself over all she read in baby-care books of the era when many claimed it did not matter whether mothers breast-fed. Tompson found she could not believe that artificial feeding could be as nutritious as the "natural way." Feeling as she did, Tompson was saddened when, after the hospital births of each of her first three children, she was told that she did not have sufficient milk and would have to put her babies on bottles. During her fourth pregnancy, destiny intervened to prevent a reoccurrence of these previous disappointments. Tompson's bent to the natural had led her to read Dr. Grantley Dick-Reed's book on natural (unmedicated) childbirth. His statistics impressed her, and she was determined that her next child would have such a birth; however, no local hospital supported the practice. Fortunately, through their involvement in the CFM, Tompson and her husband, Tommy, knew the Whites. Dr. White agreed to deliver their fourth baby at home. He also provided Tompson with the breast-feeding support she needed. Thus, she successfully nursed baby Laurel.

Although neither White nor Tompson discounted the importance of correct information as a foundation for successful nursing, both were aware that a mother needed to begin to nurse expecting to be successful. They firmly believed that the unsupportive, ill-informed, technologically oriented medical world was perpetrating an injustice on women. They were convinced that mother-to-mother help was radically different from doctor-to-mother help. It was modeling, not just verbalizing. It freed mothers to listen with their hearts, not just their minds. It began a process in which the real changes were in the way mothers saw themselves.

Bolstered by these beliefs and feelings, White and Tompson began to enlist the help of friends who had successfully nursed their infants. Edwina Froehlich vividly recalls that Tompson telephoned her the day after the picnic and declared that, although she and White had no idea how they were going to go about it, they had decided that they must start somewhere. They were planning to begin with a meeting the next week. Would Froehlich be interested? Froehlich had delayed becoming a mother until her late thirties and was then enjoying every minute of it, including breast feeding. She was very interested.

Froehlich had decided to nurse her infants for two reasons. First, since she and her siblings had all been nursed as infants, she grew up expecting to breast-feed her own children. Second, she was influenced by an experience she had while working in a Catholic action group. Through the group, she and several friends had become acquainted with an Italian priest, Father Romeo Blanchet. In discussing the American moral character, Father Blanchet had observed that most American women did not breast-feed their babies. Froehlich was both hurt and fascinated by Father Blanchet's observations. She was certain that the problem was not a lack of moral character but something else. She could remember that her older sister had been devastated by her inability to nurse and that their mother had felt herself a failure in not being able to help her daughter.

Froehlich and her friends discussed the issue at length. Some hypothesized the fast pace of American urban life caused modern women to be so busy that they were too nervous to nurse their babies. Froehlich was intrigued by the problem, even though she was single and not even committed to anyone in particular at the time. When she married, she was determined not to fall into the bottle-feeding trap. Luckily for Froehlich, her friend Father John Egan introduced her to Dr. Herbert Ratner, a great supporter of breast feeding. Ratner introduced her to his friend and protégé Dr. White. Froehlich had both Dr. White and Dr. Ratner at the foot of her bed for the birth of all her children.

With their support, Froehlich had no problem nursing her three sons. When she had nursed her infants, mothers in her apartment building sent their toddlers to watch her nurse and have the process explained to them. It made her sad to realize that being with her might be the only place these children were ever to see "what breasts are really for." Because of these experiences, White and Tompson's idea appealed to her.

Froehlich also knew someone else who she was certain would want to join. This was Viola Lennon, with whom she had been friends since they both had been involved in the Young Christian Workers (YCW), a Catholic organization for single people dedicated to bringing about social change. Lennon had also met Ratner through a priest when she was taking classes at Catholic University in 1948. By the time Lennon was expecting her first child, Ratner had become health commissioner of Oak Park, Illinois. He sent her to Dr. White, who subsequently delivered the Lennon children and gave her the help she needed to nurse them successfully. Lennon came to her first meeting out of curiosity. Simply discussing breast feeding would not have appealed to her, because nursing had gone well for her. But Froehlich had said they were going to discuss breast feeding and mothering, and mothering interested Lennon a great deal. Along with being intrigued by what she might learn at the group, Lennon believed she had something to offer as well. Her experiences in the YCW and CFM had given her an education in beginning new groups, leading meetings, and discovering the talents and skills that each person might bring to a group.

Mary White knew two other women who she thought could contribute to the new enterprise. One was her sister-in-law, Mary Ann Kerwin, who was then expecting her second child. With the Whites' help, Kerwin had nursed her first baby, so she was attracted to a plan to help other mothers in the way she had been helped. Also, as a member of the CFM, Kerwin was committed to meeting the needs of the community beyond her family. Perhaps most important, she was attracted to the idea of having discussions with other breast-feeding women with whom she could exchange information and ideas. Kerwin knew that mothers felt at a disadvantage when they tried on their own to discuss nursing diffi-culties with their doctors. She was convinced that a group of women was needed to support those who encountered problems with breast feeding.

White also telephoned Mary Ann Cahill, whom she had met through the CFM. Cahill was immediately convinced that engaging in mother-to-mother support was the right thing to do. She wished that she had received such help with her first babies. Like the other mothers, Cahill was interested in both the support the group would provide for her and the help she might give others. When White asked her whether there was anyone else who might be interested, Cahill immediately thought of Betty Wagner, because Wagner had helped her to nurse her second child successfully after she had been unable to breast-feed her first. Cahill remembers that "Betty laughed at the idea of a club for nursing mothers, but she said she'd come."[6]

GETTING IT ALL TOGETHER

The group of seven mothers met several times during the summer and early fall. They knew that if a mother was to breast-feed successfully, she must receive support early on. Otherwise, she would be likely to give up. They began their discussions by trying to pinpoint the reasons mothers foundered at breast feeding and what they needed to succeed. It was not an easy process. They brought together what seemed the most important topics. This took a while, but in time they divided the subjects into the benefits of breast feeding and old wives' tales about the practice. They held their first formal meeting in October 1956. It was attended by the seven original mothers and five of their pregnant friends. No one re-members the exact date, because they never expected to be asked for such information.

Although they would later realize that the meeting was not well orga-nized to accomplish their purpose, it was soon apparent that, even if the approach was not the best possible, it was more than adequate to en-gender enthusiasm in the women in attendance. The meeting infused the seven original mothers themselves with ever more excitement about what they had undertaken, even though they were a bit shaken as well. They wondered where they were going to get the information they needed, because there was practically nothing in print at the time. Froehlich also had another concern. Although she and the other founders were advocacy oriented, at that time their families filled their lives and kept them very busy.

Froehlich's fears were well founded. The work she and the others had begun was resonating with women in their community. Without any public announcement, the second meeting drew approximately thirty women. By the third meeting, not just friends of friends but total strangers were showing up. Not only was there a standing-room-only crowd, but many women could not even get in the door.

This response removed any vestiges of doubt that their organization was needed or that it could work. It became apparent that they could not simply proceed meeting by meeting, giving personal support. Their organization needed some formal structure, as did the information that was communicated at the meetings and through phone requests for help. It took several months of leading meetings before they arrived at an organizational structure that they sensed would best minister to the needs of mothers. That same structure has lasted until the present day. Their message, too, has remained remarkably consistent. Although the structure and the information have expanded, La Leche League's primary goal and fundamental philosophy have remained unchanged. They include not allowing the League to appear to be allied with any other cause. An early official statement reads, "People who support good mothering may reject the League if it seems to be part of another movement."[7]

The founders struggled to identify with clarity a universal message that would transcend peoples, nations, and governments and that could serve as the foundation for their philosophy. For these women, the heart of this message was that a close and happy relationship between mother and baby fostered a stronger family life for all family members. They held up the breast-feeding relationship as the model for all intrafamily relationships.

The founders defined La Leche League's goal as teaching this message to mothers because they believed that mothers formed family life. Breast feeding was both a means for achieving the kind of mothering the League espoused and a symbol of that mothering. The founders maintained that the experience of breast feeding teaches women to be better mothers and that this nurturing affects all of a mother's relationships. They had encountered mothers who had breast-fed and hated every minute of it, but they felt convinced that such mothers had focused too narrowly on the mechanics of breast feeding and not enough on good mothering through breast feeding.

The founders recognized that both breast feeding and bottle feeding could yield babies that are both emotionally and physically healthy. In fact, they did not originally intend to join the fray in the debate between the two infant-feeding methods. At the beginning they were concerned only with the fact that breast feeding had been sadly neglected. It seemed a lost art. They limited their appeal to mothers already interested in nursing who needed help to accomplish their purpose. La Leche League continues to insist that its main purpose is to help the mothers who come to them interested in breast feeding.

From the beginning, however, it has been a tightrope walk to advise mothers who wish to breast-feed without advocating breast feeding over bottle feeding. Dr. Niles Newton, a professor of behavioral sciences at Northwestern University Medical School, observed that La Leche League mothers awoke the industrial world to a value almost lost to our culture. As the organization grew and became more involved in the broader community, the perception of it as an advocacy group for breast feeding also grew. Its leaders were accused of insisting "on breast feeding when the results are negative and a qualified pediatrician recommends formula."[8]

There was some justice in these accusations. La Leche League's philosophy *was* (and is) that breast feeding is best. Its members believe that almost every mother could breast-feed if supported and well advised. League members believe the decision to breast-feed is intuitive and that it originates in a mother's heart and soul.

In focusing on good mothering through breast feeding, the founders of La Leche League were necessarily choosing to define the "good mother." Claiming that mothering is fundamentally important and that breast feeding is one of the best expressions of mothering is fundamentally different from simply saying that breast feeding is a good choice backed up by sound reasons. For League mothers, the good mother gives her baby the part of herself that is the "best" she has to give and that which the baby needs most, her milk and the comfort of her breast. Seeing how her baby depends on her, the mother recognizes that she must meet his needs.[9] For the founders, this dedication to meeting a baby's needs through breast feeding was the whole idea of loving.

There is a clear implication in these statements that mothering can be both loving and unloving. This is not, however, an assertion that bottle feeding is "nonloving" mothering. La Leche League carefully avoided such a claim. Rather, the contrast is with what Rima Apple calls "scientific motherhood." Between 1890 and 1920, there was "a significant transformation in women's idealized maternal role from the cult of domesticity [a nineteenth-century emphasis on women's special wisdom] to scientific motherhood." Scientific motherhood situated mothers in the domestic sphere. In contrast to the cult of domesticity, however, "it increasingly emphasized the importance of scientific and medical expertise" as necessary for a woman who wished to be a successful mother.[10]

League mothers distrusted reliance on expert advice over maternal instinct and mother-to-mother guidance. The earliest members of the League brought together mothers who had an interest in breast feeding so that they could give them a picture of what it meant to mother "naturally and normally" through breast feeding. Richard Frisbie, a contributing editor to *Grail* magazine, observed, "Essentially, their method is a combination of what psychologists call group therapy and plain, old-fashioned neighborly advice."[11]

The League developed an organizational structure to preserve both its philosophy and its mother-to-mother approach. In this it succeeded. At the same time, however, the intensely hierarchical nature of the organization lends itself to inflexibility of policy, and the mother-to-mother approach makes the organization vulnerable to the leader whose loyalty to League principles overruns her tact and objectivity in approaching individual mothers.

To maintain both their philosophy and the warmth of the original group, the founders, after several months of loosely structured meetings, developed a sequence of four meetings, including a fathers' meeting, to be held every three weeks. Before the year's end, the series was expanded to five. Their first manual, published in September 1958, enumerated these meetings. The first meeting pointed out the advantages of breast feeding. At the second, the mothers discussed the techniques of successful nursing. The third focused on childbirth because successful breast feeding depends in part on putting the baby to the breast as soon as he is born. For a mother to be alert enough to breast-feed immediately after her child is born, a birth in which anesthesia is not used is best. Because the idea of natural childbirth frightened many mothers, the founders felt obliged to introduce them to the basic facts and options of childbirth. They were clear that this one meeting was no substitute for childbirth classes. Rather, they offered it to stimulate mothers to consider options that would allow them to be awake after the birth. This meeting also focused on weaning and on the baby in relation to the rest of the family.

The fathers' meeting aimed to help husbands understand their wives' new roles as mothers, especially their unique and important attachments to their babies. It was important for the father to learn about these facets of new motherhood, because, at the time, men had no other source for such knowledge. The League also wanted fathers to know that the importance of the mother-baby relationship did not minimize the significance of the father's place in his child's daily care. League libraries carried an article on the importance of fathers by Newton. It demonstrated that children whose fathers had been away during their first year of life tended to be more fearful and dependent and had more difficulty in getting along with other children than did children whose fathers had been at home.[12]

This concept found a ready audience in La Leche League mothers. The founders considered inappropriate those attitudes that perceived child care and housework as women's work or that saw men who performed these tasks as "substitute mothers." They advised both parents to do what felt comfortable without worrying too much about losing their masculinity, on the one hand, or women's rights, on the other.

After using this four-meeting structure for less than a year, the group perceived a need for a meeting on nutrition. They became involved in the nutritional aspects of breast feeding when they noticed that the mothers were losing their milk because they started their babies on solid foods early. Ideas about good nutrition were fairly uninformed in the 1950s, but the founders realized that the mothers would feel better and would most likely be better mothers if they ate well.

Crystallizing the content of their meetings solved only part of the need for structure. Although the early members strove to offer correct and reasonable information, they realized that "between and around and after the words on know-how and statistics at the meetings is the *talk of the mothers about their nursing experiences.*" Moreover, these conversations had a constantly recurring theme, the understanding that the love between a nursing mother and her baby was a completely natural process that occurred gradually as the mother nursed. The strength of this conviction is illustrated by a 1960 *Chicago Tribune* article about a mother and baby whom the League supported through a major crisis. This baby had from birth suffered from severe diarrhea, breathing difficulty, and convulsive seizures because he could not tolerate any formula. With the help of La Leche League, the baby's mother was able to begin breast feeding when her son was eleven weeks old. At first, supplemental feedings of donated breast milk were necessary, but eventually he was nourished entirely by his mother's milk. La Leche League members attributed the mother's success to her own determination and resourcefulness, but the mother told the *Tribune* reporter that it was the help of the mothers who gave "so generously of their milk, their kindness, prayers, and constant encouragement" that enabled her to succeed.[13]

Because twentieth-century American mothers were drawn to "expert" advice, La Leche League felt compelled to impart sound scientific and medical facts about breast feeding. The League founders knew many mothers who had turned away reluctantly from an earlier decision to nurse because of misinformation received from doctors or hospital personnel. Even some doctors recognized that procedures in many maternity units often interfered with the management of breast feeding.[14]

As one might expect, it was difficult to present scientifically accurate information without sounding "like an advertisement for the latest drug." On receiving a letter of advice from the League, a young mother replied with the suggestion that the League put its information in everyday English instead of language so scientific that it read like an article in a medical journal. Thus, the founders became aware that technological statements about the advantages of breast feeding might not convince anyone and, indeed, might stimulate a response directed mostly at refuting the points the League had made.[15]

An additional challenge to maintaining a clear message resulted from their success. The founders set out only to help their friends who wanted to nurse their babies, but knowledge about what they were doing spread quickly beyond the confines of Franklin Park, Illinois. They began to receive so many letters and phone calls that they could not adequately respond to them by themselves. They needed written information that was both scientifically accurate and warmly written in the "natural" English requested by the young mother.

Their initial effort was a brochure. In its first printing in 1957, this pamphlet was entitled *For Better Mothers*. They quickly realized that such

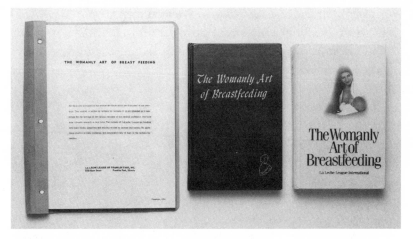

From the beginning, the founders of La Leche League found it necessary to make their advice available in published form. The 1957 edition of *The Womanly Art of Breastfeeding* was put together in loose-leaf folders. Later editions were published in book form. Each edition of the manual has gone through several printings. Not pictured here is the latest expanded version, published in 1998.

a title implied that they believed breast-feeding mothers to be better than other mothers. Having vowed to not be involved in the debate between bottle and breast feeding, they retitled the brochure *Your Baby and You.* If the first title was too judgmental, this one was too vague. The third edition was entitled more specifically *Why Nurse Your Baby?* All three editions imparted the same information, but the third, printed in 1959 after the League had crystallized its philosophy, included a paragraph entitled "Mothering Is Our Objective."

A short pamphlet rapidly proved unequal to the task of responding to all the questions that poured in. Although the founders, all of whom had young families to claim most of their time and attention, were making no attempt to parlay their success into an elaborate organization, their resolve was being overcome by reality. The founders decided to write and publish a manual. It was printed on 8½-by-11-inch sheets, which were put together in loose-leaf folders from the local variety store. Over the next five years, seventeen thousand copies of this first edition of the manual were sold. Every copy was accompanied by a personal letter from one of the founders, who felt that however beneficial and valuable the manual was, it would never replace the most important thing La Leche offered, mother-to-mother support. Meanwhile, Marian Tompson developed a newsletter for the organization. Its purpose was to supplement the basic information available through the manual by keeping mothers in touch with one another through personal stories. The newsletter filled a major void because few mothers had anyone in their circle of friends who was breast feeding.

The first issue appeared in May 1958. In order to meet their responsibilities, the founders had to drop all activities outside the League. However, they were careful that their families remained the first priority in their lives. Marian Tompson wrote in the second issue of the *La Leche League News*, "We regret that this issue of the *NEWS* is reaching you a few weeks late. But a siege of the regular measles at our house — with five children succumbing at one time — topped off with father's case of blood poisoning, naturally got first priority."[16] The sense that she was first and foremost a mother never left Tompson.

From these beginnings, La Leche League's publications grew both in number and in the range of materials. The League also endorsed many other publications, including the 596-page *You Can Breastfeed Your Baby—Even in Special Situations*. Its author, Dorothy Brewster, claimed that there are very few circumstances under which a woman who wants to breast-feed cannot do so.[17] The loose-leaf version of the manual was replaced by a printed expanded version in 1958. This manual went through eleven printings before a third edition was published, in 1981, to cover expanding knowledge and concerns. In 1998, a fourth edition was published. This edition brings mothers the latest in scientific findings about breast feeding but remains eminently readable.

With the publication of the manual and the newsletter, La Leche League settled on a basic structure for communicating its philosophy. Realizing that letters and literature could never substitute adequately for a direct mother-to-mother approach, however, the founders were determined to find a way for new groups to function independently of the groups they themselves attended. They kept this new outreach simple because they preferred to spend their time helping mothers, not overseeing an organizational structure. In the beginning, when the League grew slowly, they simply handled the overflow crowds by splitting into two groups. As the League flourished, however, new methods to deal with its success would be required.

In 1958, three Chicago mothers who had attended several meetings in Franklin Park suggested they start a group for their neighbors. Around that same time, a woman in Cleveland heard about the League and wrote to ask to start a group there. Less than a year and a half after the first meeting, the number of groups had quadrupled. This process continued without any formal control. By 1962 the founders became concerned over this lack of formality when they discovered that many groups using their name did not adhere to the mothering philosophy around which they centered their basic concepts. Also, some leaders were being tactless and uncaring in their dealings with pregnant women or new mothers, a practice that conflicted with League policy. La Leche League stressed that when a mother requested help in solving some difficulty, the goal was to help her look at her unique baby and discover possible reasons for the difficulty. It was vital to avoid telling the mother what to do according to some general principle. The particular nursing problem might be connected with unalterable circumstances in that family.[18]

The founders realized that they were going to have to put a stop to overzealousness and non-League attitudes toward mothering. To do so, they developed a process for qualifying leaders. Mary Jane Brizzolara, one of the League's earliest members, was given the job of qualifying leaders. Her goal was to maintain the feeling of "coming home" that she had experienced at her first La Leche League meeting. She aimed for quality control to maintain the standards and philosophy that the League had started out with and to be certain that new leaders were giving out correct breast-feeding information.

Brizzolara's original approach was to send questionnaires to prospective leaders. They were returned to Franklin Park, read, and sent back to the women with suggestions for additional readings. Eventually, if a woman agreed to the League's attitude toward mothering, she was certified as an official La Leche League leader.

As the League grew, it became impossible for the Franklin Park new group chairperson to guide every new leader through this process. In 1964, when Marybeth Doucette became new group chairperson, she made two important changes. She required a résumé as part of the approval process, and she established new group chairpersons for any state that had a large number of women applying for leadership. By 1972, every state had such an officer. Local leaders took the initial steps in guiding a mother toward leadership. Leaders were advised to be certain that those who represented the League genuinely embraced its ideals. The League handbook also cautioned, however, "Of course, we all fall short occasionally, usually for good and understandable reasons, but we also, hopefully, keep learning and maturing."[19]

To aid leaders in nurturing applicants, the League developed an application packet. Any leader in a group might use the packet, but ordinarily the leader who had known the applicant longest oversaw the process through which the applicant became a leader. At every stage, the emphasis was to keep the warmth of the mother-to-mother approach within the effort to maintain quality control. In evaluating the applicant the leader was asked to be certain the applicant's philosophy adhered to the League's, she understood the responsibilities of leadership, she evidenced a warmth and concern toward other mothers in the group, she was familiar with League literature, and she had grown in mothering since coming to meetings. It was the leader's responsibility to decide whether the application process would continue past the first stages.[20] Understanding the weight of this responsibility, new group chairpersons stayed in close contact with leaders during the process. Illinois's new group chairperson, Barbara King, wrote to a leader in Chicago, "I appreciate the time you are giving to Martha to help her grow into leadership." After detailing her concerns and urging the leader to call with concerns of her own, she added, "Hope you and your family are well. Getting ready for spring?"[21] An evaluation letter written about "Martha" was highly enthusiastic and personal but tackled negatives as well: "Although she did feel that her own approach to good nutrition was more stringent than the League's, she could see mothers needed to be helped to change their family's eating habits gradually."[22]

Leader applicants were also encouraged to become a part of the group process even before being certified, as they were understood to be vital in promoting La Leche League warmth and friendliness. Leaders encouraged mother/applicants to introduce themselves to newcomers and to help mothers of crying babies understand that it happened to everyone. Another way an applicant could help the League was by projecting a good image at meetings. League literature urged them to remember that League suggestions were only guidelines. Leaders reminded them to nurse discreetly at meetings, since indiscreet nursing could offend a newcomer. Also, open discussion of weaning ages was discouraged, as it might upset new mothers.[23]

Along with formalizing the League structure at the group level, the early members of La Leche League also found it necessary to develop a structure to oversee the ever-expanding organization. Another important task was to define the League's relationship to the medical community.

Before the founders had even held their first meeting for other mothers, they had informally formed a board of officers with Marian Tompson as the president. By the time the League was a year old, the board began meeting regularly. At first these meetings centered around group business, how to handle unusual nursing situations, and the content of the meetings. As more women became involved in these decision-making meetings, their size grew until it became necessary in 1962 to divide the League geographically into smaller sections that were called chapters. Each chapter could then have its own board. The founders came to be known as the executive board. This reorganization allowed them to focus their attention on policy. Free of the day-to-day responsibilities that now fell to individual chapters, the board met as often as necessary to determine policy and to administer the overall organization.

By the early 1960s the founders of the League, which was originally incorporated in 1958 as La Leche League of Franklin Park, sensed a need for a name that would reflect the organization's growing scope of influence. On June 2, 1964, the name was officially changed to La Leche League International, Inc. By that time, 115 groups in the United States and six groups abroad were affiliated with the League.

When the League's first national convention was held in 1964, 425 mothers and 100 babies attended it. The founders realized there was a need to formalize the connection between the individual groups and the international organization. The executive board created the position of executive coordinator. The coordinator, in turn, appointed a coordinator for each state because chapter coordinators could no longer handle all the work in their geographic area.

As each state coordinator was selected, she began writing a leader's newsletter. These letters were of primary importance because they clarified and amplified League philosophy for the individual leaders. When disputes and questions arose over issues such as the introduction of solids, the coordinator, through the newsletter, could be sure the League's policy was well understood. In addition, the coordinator oversaw each group in the state by reviewing a report for every meeting held in the state. Soon, however, the number of groups outstripped the state coordinators' ability to meet the needs of every group adequately. The idea of reducing the number of reports to one each series was rejected because it left the coordinators feeling out of touch with the groups. To solve these problems, assistant state coordinators were appointed. Eventually even this arrangement was inadequate. Ohio faced this crisis first. When the number of groups in the state reached one hundred, the Ohio League organized a system of districts within the state. Eventually other states would follow Ohio's lead.

After the official change of names to La Leche League International, Inc., had taken effect, a committee was established at the League's headquarters in Franklin Park to oversee the expanding organization. Each member of this committee was responsible for a certain number of states. These women both advised the state coordinators and helped develop the League as an international organization. At first, they also oversaw the certification of new leaders, but in 1973 a new position, chairman of leader applications, evolved. These chairpersons handled the application procedure at the district level.

Although it was important to maintain control over the organization, another basic principle also inspired this increase in the number of positions: a mother's first priority was always her family. Thus, no one mother should ever take on more responsibility than she could handle. One coordinator reminded her leaders, "Don't ever lose sight of LLL goals. Husbands, families, babies must always come first; then we can do our best for LLL."[24] In 1967, *Leaven*, the leaders' newsletter, asked various leaders what they felt was the best benefit of being a League leader. The Illinois leader and editor of the *La Leche League News*, Rosemary Fahey, replied, "Another baby has now arrived and I just want to look at her and feed her and watch her grow for a while. Of all the organizations which I have ever worked for, LLL is the only one which accepts this as a reasonable excuse."[25]

As La Leche League has grown, two aspects have remained unchanged. League leaders continue to put family needs ahead of League responsibilities, and the international organization continues to maintain control over information and procedures. In 1981, Mary White stated, "We want to do our best to see that our principles and policies are upheld wherever the League is represented. This will help preserve the unity in La Leche around the world." She also noted, "The very fact that so many different peoples are involved in our work means there will always be a refreshing diversity of approaches to mothering through breastfeeding . . . probably as many as there are mothers and babies."[26] Unfortunately, the

League has not always been able to inspire every leader with this same refreshing openness.

BETWEEN MOTHER AND DOCTOR: BRIDGING THE GAP

Although the founders of La Leche League held that medical misinformation was often responsible for a mother's failure to breast-feed, they never intended for the League to function independently of the medical community or to compete with it. The League has always depended on medical advisors. The first of these advisors were Drs. Ratner and White. It would be difficult to overestimate the significance of Ratner's contributions to the League. He edited *Child and Family Digest*, which was essential reading to the founders. It was from Ratner that the League received its faith in the family as the foundation of a healthy society and its concern that the family was in crisis. It was also from him and from White that they gained the courage to set about righting this situation, even if only in a small way. White's most important contribution to League philosophy was his belief that hospitals and doctors were the secondary, not the primary, caretakers of the sick child. White was reluctant to prescribe an antibiotic if he was not certain that rest and quiet might not work as well. He avoided hospitalizing a sick child whenever possible. He endorsed keeping the child at home in an atmosphere he believed to be more healing than hospitals. He preferred to deliver babies at home, seeing childbirth as an experience to be cherished, not an ordeal to be endured. He saw his role as helping mothers realize their importance, not just within the family but within the world as well.

Both Ratner and White saw the League as supportive of the medical community, not as a threat to it. Ratner noted that League leaders relied on the continuing supervision of physicians. From his viewpoint, leaders served as assistants to the medical profession in the goal of achieving the optimum nurturing of newborns. White was convinced of the health benefits of nursing for mother and baby. Yet, he knew that he had often failed to persuade mothers to nurse. He observed that League mothers were more successful than he was because they dispensed information as part of mother-to-mother dialogue.

La Leche League depended on the help and encouragement of doctors and supported the medical community in its work. The founders recognized that, with so few doctors supporting breast feeding, it was important to join hands with those who did. Their knowledge and experience were vital aids to developing League expertise. After inviting Dr. E. Robbins Kimball, pediatrician and head of the Evanston Milk Bank, to talk to the board in 1958, the founders asked him to become an advisor to the League. Later, Marian Tompson heard Dr. Robert Mendelsohn speak, recognized him as a kindred soul, and invited him to a medical advisors' meeting. In quick succession, several other doctors joined. The League sought out specialists in jaundice, immunology, allergies, emotional needs, and natural childbirth. In 1971, the board's name was changed to the Professional Advisory Board because some of its members were not medical doctors. This board was central to the functioning of the League. The founders were aware that without the credibility and acceptability afforded them by the board, parents might have been wary of their advice. It was not an era attuned to women's wisdom.

Because of the League's growth and its increasing need to communicate with medical professionals, the board developed a professional liaison department to communicate with them. This department served two functions: to help the professional community understand League principles and to help League leaders communicate effectively with medical professionals. The department also asked that leaders report instances of especially good rapport with local doctors, including times when they had been able to convert a potentially difficult situation into one of friendly cooperation.[27]

In spite of these steps, individual leaders still worried about mothers who received medical advice that conflicted with the League's advice and were often tempted to directly contradict advice given by a local doctor when the leader was convinced that it was mistaken. But the editors of the *Leader's Handbook*, Judy Kahel and Lorrie Dyal, insisted it was always a mistake to argue with a physician on a professional level.[28] To avoid antagonizing local physicians by appearing to overstep their role, Mendelsohn suggested that local groups attempt to develop a close relationship with the medical associations in their area.[29]

As the League grew, however, relying solely upon local leaders to educate doctors in their area proved to be inefficient. Longtime leader Vera Turton proposed that the League provide a program for which doctors might receive accreditation. The American Medical Association (AMA) agreed to survey a seminar for physicians presented by the

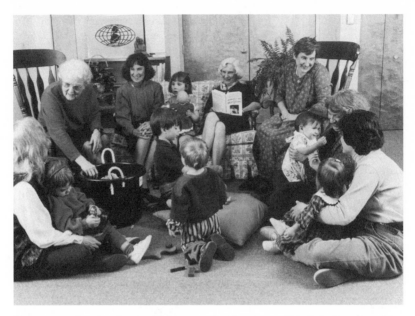

Forty years after they began the League, the founders still find their greatest joy
in gathering to share parenting stories with young mothers and their babies.

League to see whether it could be accredited. With the help of several
members of the Professional Advisory Board, the League was able to
create its first Physicians' Breastfeeding Seminar in 1973. Only provi-
sional accreditation was granted, because the AMA was concerned about
the League's small budget, but the evaluation forms filled out by doctors
who attended that first seminar and subsequent ones attested to the
League's effectiveness. The seminar led one hospital to change the entire
organization of its nursery. In another case, a Michigan doctor hired La
Leche League leaders as breast-feeding counselors. These seminars continue today.

Also continuing today is a program that was inspired by that doctor in
Michigan, the Lactation Consultant Program, which is an education
program similar to the workshops that the League runs for physicians
and other medical personnel. It differs in that its purpose is to train
women to act as professional lactation consultants. After being certified
through the League program, these women can work in conjunction
with physicians, hospitals, or clinics. They can also develop a one-on-one
practice with individual breast-feeding mothers. Some consultants are
former League leaders, whereas others come from the medical commu-

nity. Like leaders, they strive to help get the breast-feeding relationship off to a good start and to be there when difficulties arise. Unlike leaders, they charge for their services and are not involved in La Leche League's many outreach programs.

SPEAKING IN TONGUES:
THE MANY LANGUAGES OF LA LECHE LEAGUE

La Leche League perceives these many facets of its organization — the mother-to-mother approach, the carefully constructed hierarchy, and its partnership with the medical community — as the heart of its success. Yet, beyond these factors lie several other, less-well-known facets of the League. They also contribute to its extraordinary persuasiveness and account for the fact that its philosophy has been embraced by hundreds of professionals and millions of parents over the short span of its existence.

The organization is the bearer of a particular strain of practical rationality within which is incorporated highly powerful religious meanings. The tradition of practical reason has its origins in Aristotle's concept of *phronesis*. Reason as *phronesis* asks the questions "What should we do?" and "How should we live?" La Leche League's practical wisdom is presented via an interaction between a persuasive practice and a multidimensional language. For the League, this language has its roots in efforts to counter what its members considered scientific misinformation with scientific information. The League's use of scientific language is, however, only one aspect of its wisdom, and even this aspect contains within it references to the basic religious foundation of La Leche League language. La Leche League draws on certain developmental psychologies to explicate its theory of moral obligation, but it is Catholic natural law theory that undergirds that theory.

The League's particular practical wisdom shares in some important aspects the practical wisdom of the American Catholic Church, the faith community of all the founders. The practical reasoning goes beyond Catholicism, however, to include the broader spectrum of American religious thinking that has also contributed to League philosophy. La Leche League exercises its practical wisdom so effectively because its narratives contain the power of implicit religious symbols and convictions. These symbols and convictions render its moral ideals appealing to those who have internalized an awe of the Divine Mother, the symbol of which in Catholicism is Mary, the mother of Jesus.[30] This symbol finds expression in most great religious traditions the world over. In addition, although Americans may not see mothers as gods, they certainly tend to see them as saints.

League language is made even more complex because, while much of its explicit expression is antifeminist, its perception of what it means to be a woman can be understood to be implicitly feminist in its origins. Indeed, this perception stands in stark contrast to traditional Catholicism and coheres amazingly easily with contemporary Catholic feminism, although never as a perfect match.

The next seven chapters will detail this interweaving of languages. A final chapter will explore how the League's practical wisdom interacts with contemporary realities. Because the League's wisdom has developed within a tradition of practical reason, it has the ability to change as it confronts the shifts within family life in the late twentieth century. The organization's theory of moral obligation is strong enough to include a more complex understanding of women's roles in the community without compromising its primary ethical concern with meeting the needs of infants and children. Although the League will be shown to be more flexible than is often perceived, its own failure to grasp the full depth of its religious metaphors and theories of moral obligation has engendered a degree of rigidity. A more open exploration of these implicit metaphors will demonstrate that La Leche League praxis could offer more options for today's or tomorrow's families than does either the League's traditional ideology or any other theories of women's roles within the family.[31] This possibility depends on the League's ability to acknowledge its roots in religious meanings, give them their fullest expression, and, thus, save them from sentimentalization by secular forces.

chapter 2

· ·

Mothers, Medicine,
and Misinformation

When the founding mothers of La Leche League formed their first group, they had two firm goals in mind. First, they wanted to replace with correct information the misinformation that mothers hoping to breast-feed often received from their doctors. Second, they wished to offer mother-to-mother support that doctors could not give to expectant or new mothers. The League succeeded in these goals, in part, because their knowledge of breast feeding was and remains excellent and because their support techniques fell solidly within the realm of nonmedical healing. As Jerome Frank states in *Persuasion and Healing: A Comparative Study of Psychotherapy*, this form of healing involves interplay between patient, healer, and group. It serves to help the patient harmonize her inner conflicts within a frame of reference that integrates her with the group, stirs her emotionally, combats her demoralization, and strengthens her self-confidence.[1] Information and technique alone, however, do not account for the League's wide-ranging success. Just as important is the understanding that God is both personal and good and that God's material creation — that is, Nature — is also good. From this metaphor flows an understanding of human tendencies and needs as created morally good by God and, therefore, a central source of moral obligation.

Thus, when we compare the League's approach to infant care with that of the medical community, we see two opposing understandings of what should be the source of information about the common good as it related to infant care and nutrition. For many in the medical community, the health of the infant depended on physicians taking the control of babies and children away from old women and uneducated nurses and making certain that children were placed under the care of physicians, whether they were healthy or ill.[2]

For the founders of La Leche League, the foundation for a healthy mother-baby couple was breast feeding. Breast feeding meant a link to other mothers and a sign of womanly power. It was a miracle, belonging rightfully to mothers, babies, and families everywhere. Thus, the debate involved every dimension of practical moral reasoning. First, the medical community and the League relied on conflicting concepts about the source of the common good. For the medical community, it was scientific and technical progress. For La Leche League, it was nature abetted by tradition. Second, their ethical first principles conflicted because a great gulf existed between their definitions of the infant's basic human needs. Doctors did not place nearly as great an emphasis on mother-baby proximity as did the League. Third, the doctors and League members also differed over the social context of child care, medically dependent versus medically assisted. In addition, each group interpreted differently the doctor's role regarding the family, the mother's relationship to her doctor and to her child, and the father's place within the family.

League information is derived from two main sources, the biological and human sciences and the personal experiences of mothers. Both of these sources carry powerful worldviews, and both are incorporated into League ideology, creating a powerful quasi-religious force within the organization. This is not to say that the information is incorrect, but only that its persuasiveness does not rely solely on its scientific veracity or on the warmth and empathy of League members.

SCIENTIFIC MOTHERHOOD

"Scientific motherhood" is a term Rima Apple, author of *Mothers and Medicine*, used to designate a coherent ideology that developed in the late nineteenth and early twentieth centuries and that "increasingly emphasized the importance of scientific and medical expertise to the development of proper childbearing techniques."[3] Although women continued to be children's primary care providers, both they and the medical community believed that they needed expert advice to perform their duties successfully. Most members of the medical community believed that science alone could find the answers to the crisis in infant health. Medical practitioners perceived human existence as deeply haunted by the chaotic ravages of disease and human ignorance, which they felt obliged to defeat. Such understandings contrasted profoundly with La Leche League's reliance on an all-knowing, all-caring Providence as a guide to moral obligations.

By the time of the founding of La Leche League, medically supervised breast feeding was well established. Dr. Lawrence Gartner, chairman of the pediatrics department at the University of Chicago School of Medicine, has gathered two thousand years of medical advice on breast feeding. Through his research, he has learned that from era to era and culture to culture there has been considerable consistency in the vocabulary used in such advice. In the Western world in particular, there has been a long tradition that holds that physicians, not mothers, are the experts in infant feeding. Gartner points out that often this advice was the very opposite of what would today be understood as good management of breast feeding. Since the second century, physicians have advised women to delay breast feeding for various lengths of time after birth. There was also widespread belief that the first milk to flow out of the breast should not be given to the infant. One fifteenth-century textbook advised feeding newborns solids before allowing them to nurse. Physicians worried about overfeeding the baby, and there were mechanical devices for emptying the breast. Doctors vacillated between the opposing beliefs that illness could be carried via the milk to the baby and that mother's milk was a cure for certain illnesses. Interestingly, Gartner also found a consistent belief in the psychological benefits of breast feeding that mirrors today's perspectives. He further found that physicians have expressed a common horror over the practice of wet nursing in ancient China, in sixteenth-century Germany and France, and in eighteenth-century England. Not only did they believe that wet nurses might be a source of illness, but they worried that the infant might lose its affection for its mother.[4]

Although the perception that physicians were experts in infant feeding did not arise in the twentieth century, it increased then. Even though nineteenth-century medical advice on breast feeding was not always adequate, until late in that century most doctors believed that mother's milk was the best infant food and urged mothers to nurse their own infants.

As research on infant mortality accumulated in the last quarter of the nineteenth century, however, many physicians began to turn their attentions to this question in earnest. Dr. T. B. Greenley felt compelled to act to stem the tragic tide of infant deaths. In 1889, Greenley wrote that the statistics presented doctors with the question of what they, "as sanitarians, philanthropists and medical men," might do to modify or curtail the infant mortality rate.[5] Greenley saw little hope in instructing the poor in large cities about the benefits of breast feeding, since they lived where "squalor, filth and degradation" prevailed over "cleanliness and good morals." He also rued that trend of mothers "in good or ordinary health, who, for the sake of enjoying fashionable life or for any other selfish motive" chose not to breast-feed. He believed that they were guilty not only of "a sin against true motherhood" but also of "possible, unintentional infanticide." Greenley felt that these reasons necessitated a close supervision over young children by physicians.[6]

Many other physicians also believed that a mother's behavior and diet seriously affected the quality of her milk, and since they had low expectations that mothers would engage in healthy practices during or after pregnancy, they tended to expect that mothers would be unable to nurse their children. One doctor, J. A. Work, claimed, "Many parents do not even have instinct as to feeding their young that the lower order of animals have." Work believed that these parents were completely ignorant of the benefits of breast feeding and that they fed infants anything they themselves enjoyed. He found even the use of cow's-milk formula suspect because parents tended to feed their infants an indeterminate amount of milk on a totally unregulated schedule. Work thought the mothers he observed lacked natural affection for their infants. Believing that fewer than a third of infants were actually wanted by their parents, he maintained that a good artificial formula was necessary because "fashionable mothers" did not want their "liberties infringed upon" and many poor mothers deserted their progeny to foundling homes.[7]

This perception of mothers as ignorant and uncaring may explain why physician E. A. Wood asked, "What is the best substitute for human milk?" rather than, "How can we help mothers become successful breast-feeders?" Wood believed that mothers' ignorance caused them to feed their babies milk that was unfit for any purpose. The unfitness of the milk he blamed on vendors, holding that they were veritable murderers. Wood urged his fellow physicians to focus on developing an appropriate and sanitary infant formula as a major step in preventive health care.[8]

Therefore, a number of research-oriented physicians devoted themselves to improving substitutes for human milk. By the 1880s, the substitutes developed by these doctors were manufactured commercially. Advertising in women's magazines, doctors offered consumers free samples of their products and booklets on infant feeding that gave the scientific rationale for their breast-milk substitute. Despite the fact that infant feeding was a very small part of medical practice in the 1870s and 1880s, infant-food companies cultivated medical patronage.

The breast-milk substitutes succeeded so well that the weight of the discussion in the infant nutrition field was directed toward determining the best alternative to mother's milk. Women themselves were swept into this discussion. They wrote letters of advice to each other and articles for women's journals. These writings acknowledged women's evolving doubt about the adequacy of breast feeding and their growing knowledge of bottle feeding. Concerns with helping each other successfully breast-feed faded into the background.

This passing of the guidance of infant care out of the domestic sphere and into the scientific sphere reflected American culture at the turn of the century. Scientific knowledge held a privileged status. The rather ambiguous term "science" had become practically synonymous with progress and reform. Physicians stressed a close identity between science and medicine. They emphasized that they were experts who held knowledge unavailable to those outside their profession. This claim generated an ever-widening gulf between physicians and mothers. Doctors endeavored to replace traditional maternal knowledge with the latest scientific discoveries. With each ensuing decade, more and more mothers turned away from information given by female relatives, neighbors, and friends and became increasingly dependent on the guidance of "scientific experts — namely, the physicians."[9]

Formula feeding as a subject for research and intense discussion intrigued these scientifically oriented physicians in a way that mother-centered breast feeding did not. When Dr. T. M. Rotch addressed the

Pan-American Medical Congress held in Washington, D.C., in September 1893, he acknowledged that traditionally the average human breast-fed infant was more likely to survive than were infants fed by any other method. In spite of this fact, Rotch went on to claim that science could discover those elements in breast milk that made it the best-known infant food. He declared that when scientists "laid bare by the search-light of patient and laborious investigation" all these elements, then they would be able to produce a breast-milk substitute that was not subject to the vagaries of what he called maternal "nervous disturbance or improper living."[10]

Unfortunately, a truly healthy substitute for mother's milk was not developed until well into the twentieth century. While the experts focused on developing the best artificial substitute for breast milk rather than on overcoming any problem mothers experienced in attempting to nurse their babies, many infants died of inadequate nutrition. In many cities, more than one-third of all infants died before their fifth birthday. Realizing that the infant mortality rate could be linked to the inadequate nutrition in commercial infant foods, pediatricians focused on bringing the distribution of infant foods more directly under their control. Although they believed that anyone who had the care of an infant needed medical advice on its feeding, the physicians did not hold that infant care should be completely directed by medical research. Rather, they were convinced that everyday medical practice and years of experience were just as important as chemical research. In fact, often the practitioners depended on basic cow's-milk mixtures that they themselves modified according to their experience. Still, like the researchers, these practitioners did not believe that nursing alone could assure an infant's health if the mother were not under the strict supervision of the physician.

Unaware of the natural antibiotic properties in breast milk, but with an increasing awareness that human milk was important to infant health, medical professionals continued to use human milk as the standard for any substitute infant food.[11] At the same time, however, they continued to hold that the degree to which conditions could affect a mother's milk was such that maternal nursing did not assure that the infant received the most healthful nutriment. What they did learn from studying mother's milk was that from one time to another during the baby's first year, the exact combination of fat, protein, and sugar in the milk varied. Therefore, they sought to develop an infant food that could adjust to the baby's needs. This approach meant the doctors' examinations of the baby could best determine when these adjustments might be required. The differences in advice between individual doctors was so great that their clients — the mothers — were often confused, especially when their doctors recommended a complicated formula they had to prepare at home. Manufacturers of infant food took advantage of this dissatisfaction and stressed their own scientific respectability. Increasingly, formula manufacturers convinced medical professionals, as well as parents, that their formula was the best and most practical solution to the problems of infant feeding. By the 1920s, physicians accepted that infants who were bottle-fed with medical supervision compared favorably with breast-fed infants in terms of weight gain, growth, and morbidity.[12]

By the middle decades of the twentieth century, physicians, while not denying that "good" breast milk was the best infant food, agreed that formula was fully adequate if the need to wean should arise. One physician even suggested, "Failure of a baby to gain on a well-balanced formula does not necessarily imply that the formula per se is at fault, and it certainly should not be considered an indication to change to something else."[13] Somewhat earlier in the century, the apparent good health of most formula-fed infants had moved practitioners from the conviction that bottle feeding could healthfully augment or replace breast feeding to a belief that, in many instances, artificial feeding could have positive benefits for infant health. In 1931, an editorial in the *Journal of the American Medical Association* claimed that "breast feeding has become irksome if not actually difficult for many mothers of the present generation. There is considerable cheer, therefore, in the increasing evidence that artificial feeding can be made far more safe and satisfactory than seemed to be the case in former times."[14]

As bottle feeding became less complex, it gained more acceptance. Also, as more was learned about the composition of breast milk, researchers felt more and more confident claiming that their formula approximated breast milk. Practitioners also liked the fact that if a baby reacted badly to a formula, they could alter its makeup. Mother's milk, which modifies itself, was out of their control. The disadvantages and shortcomings of breast feeding were now considered in choosing an infant-feeding method. Ironically, dietary supplements discovered necessary for formula-fed babies were sometimes considered necessary for breast-fed infants as well. Orange juice for vitamin C and cod liver oil for vitamin D were regularly added to their diet.

The physicians passed their fascination with the chemistry of milk on to the mothers, who were also fascinated and comforted by this "scientific" approach. The doctors feared that without a physician's regular oversight, not only infant feeding but also all other aspects of child care would be mishandled by women. They stressed the need for the continuing education of mothers by their medical advisors. From this desire, a paradox arose: doctors wished mothers to be "scientific" in their approach, but they did not wish mothers to feel so well educated in child care that they did not turn to their physicians for guidance. Practitioners sincerely believed that replacing the old tradition of woman-to-woman education with the physician-to-mother approach had saved literally thousands of lives, so to prevent future childhood mortality and morbidity, women must not take child care into their own hands again.

By midcentury, mothers were more frequently making an initial choice for bottle feeding, and "most practitioners believed that if a mother did not wish to breast feed her infant, then the doctor should accept her decision, since most babies, even newborns, did well with bottle feeding that was medically directed."[15] This belief in the efficacy of bottle feeding also encouraged doctors to be less than supportive of the mothers who wished to breast-feed but were having problems. On the other hand, one physician, Frank Richardson, feared that the emphasis on the physician's role in supervising the bottle-fed infant might be construed as eliminating the role the physician plays in breast feeding. He wrote, "To be sure, the breast-fed baby may well require fewer medical visits than his bottle-fed brother. But if he is to remain breast-fed, he ought to be kept under the surveillance of his doctor at least during the first half year of his life. Otherwise, his mother's milk may suddenly cease to be an apparently inexhaustible fountain."[16]

Thus, even physicians who advocated breast feeding supported a dependence on expert advice. Undoubtedly, the change from the practice of only ill infants being brought to doctors to routine well-baby care saved thousands of young lives. Richardson's confidence that a physician's advice would serve as the foundation for continued breast feeding was, however, not borne out in reality.

In retrospect, we can appraise the situation as a failure of communication. Physicians were highly trained in medical science. They approached the problem of infant mortality using reason and scientific research, but they made no careful attempt to integrate this perspective with the knowledge and experience of those who struggled day in and day out with the life-threatening diseases of infancy, the mothers.

Physicians, in most instances, treated infants who were not thriving. When breast feeding succeeded, mothers were less likely to seek a physician's advice. Thus, the reasons they were successful were not apparent to most doctors. An authentic communication between "experts" and participants could not occur until women who wished to breast-feed attained a more self-assured position in the public realm.

BREAST FEEDING AND THE "EXPERTS"

As the twentieth century progressed, mothers were turning increasingly for guidance to child-care manuals. One of the most popular of these was L. Emmett Holt's *The Care and Feeding of Children*. This book went through twelve revisions, seventy-five printings, and translations into Spanish, Russian, and Chinese. It remained popular from the time of its first publication in 1894 well into the 1940s. Holt's uncompromising adherence to hygiene for the prevention of infection led him to advocate strictly regimented feeding patterns. He also advised against holding infants any more than was absolutely necessary. Both of these procedures undermine successful breast feeding. Another well-read manual on child care was H. L. Mencken's *What You Ought to Know about Your Baby*. Mencken based his advice on Holt's approach. Although his manual lacked the scope of Holt's book, it displayed a lively, humorous style that made for easy reading. It was published through the first three decades of the century.[17] Toward the midcentury, physicians began to question some tenets of this rigid approach but without overcoming those aspects of Holt's method that interfered with successful breast feeding.

Dr. Benjamin Spock was a pediatrician and popular child-care expert during the years the founding mothers were raising their children. The publication of his *Common Sense Book of Baby and Child Care* in 1946 made Spock *the* baby doctor for a generation of children. The book covered five hundred topics. By 1985, Spock's book had gone through four editions and had sold over thirty million copies in thirty-eight languages. His approach was considerably more relaxed than Holt's. He had confidence that the adaptability of parents and infants meant that parents could learn to meet their infant's needs without following rigid regimens laid down by a pediatrician. His approach to breast feeding, as well as that of other midcentury pediatricians, however, was not informed enough to help the mother whose breast-feeding experience had begun poorly. Because the philosophy of Spock and like-minded pediatricians guided many parents in the same era in which La Leche League was founded, it was often the advice against which the League had to contend. Like many pediatricians of his time, Spock upheld the principle that breast feeding had definite known advantages. He also encouraged mothers who wished to breast-feed to do so, but two aspects of his advice undercut this encouragement. First, many of his suggestions were more likely to end than to prolong the breast-feeding experience. Second, he readily accepted that if breast feeding presented problems, no physical or emotional loss to baby or mother resulted in switching the infant to the bottle. Thus, a trend toward this more relaxed approach to parenting in the midcentury did little to arrest the erosion of breast feeding as the preferred choice for infant nutrition.

Thus, from the late nineteenth until well past the mid-twentieth century, misinformed "expert advice" undermined rather than advanced the breast-feeding experience. Spock's advice, like that of many of his contemporary practitioners, was the opposite of what La Leche League would advise in a similar case. Eight aspects of such misinformation stand out. First, many physicians minimized the value of breast feeding. They made little of the differences between breast and bottle feeding. Spock *began* his chapter on breast feeding with a litany of its disadvantages. Bottle feeding, he stated, was easier than breast feeding because the mother is free to come and go and can measure with certainty the amount of milk her baby receives. Spock also expressed concern over the adverse affects breast feeding might have on the mother's physical health. While suggesting that mothers eat according to their appetite, he held that breast feeding was "exhausting and should be stopped if the mother is losing weight that she can't afford to lose." These two pieces of advice seemed to conflict and would certainly be confusing to a new mother. In a clear acceptance of the medical expert's role in such a case, however, he insisted, "The mother's doctor is the one to decide." As to the baby's physical health, Spock downplayed the advantages, claiming that protection against disease through breast feeding had never been proved.[18] In contrast, Vernal Packard, like many other physicians, acknowledged the immunological advantages of breast milk, but he believed that through research immunological agents could be built into formula. He believed that they would offer better protection against bacteria and viruses than could mother's milk.[19] Whereas Spock accepted that nursing was a psychologically healthy experience for the mother, he was less assured of the benefits to the baby. Dr. Lendon Smith's doubts were more outspoken. He claimed that many babies were upset when held. "These babies just do not want to be touched and handled when they are eating — it is too distracting."[20] Spock argued strongly that bottle feeding could be as medically safe and as emotionally satisfying for mother and baby as breast feeding. Keeping in close touch with the doctor was the best guarantor of the baby's continuing health, whether it was breast or bottle fed. In *The Politics of Breastfeeding*, Gabrielle Palmer pointed out the irony of this position. She wrote, "On one hand there is eagerness to claim that artificially-fed babies are just as healthy as breastfed ones; on the other hand, there is an obsessive desire to imitate human milk, and it is used as the 'gold standard' to sell the commercial product."[21]

Physicians typically accommodated not only hospital routines but also whatever expectations about breast feeding mothers brought with them. Dr. Howard Markel emphasized that, while physicians may hold that breast feeding is the healthier choice, they must also realize that they have entered into a "partnership of two equals" with the mother whose choice of feeding method must be honored without pressure from the doctor to choose breast feeding.[22]

Spock noted that many mothers would not even consider breast feeding because bottle feeding was the custom and seemed the natural choice to them. For such women, breast feeding went against the grain. Spock held that this deeply held revulsion against nursing should be accommodated.[23] The antipathy toward breast feeding has a long history. Robert Boostrom noted that long before bottle feeding, mothers who could afford to do so avoided nursing their infants. He speculated that this rejection was related to embarrassment about sexuality.[24] D. B. Jelliffe believed this revulsion might have increased in this century as the breast moved from having a "mixed nurturing and sexual role to one of primary erotic significance."[25] Even proponents of breast feeding recognized this as a serious and sometimes insurmountable problem. Karen Pryor, an advocate of breast feeding and author of *Nursing Your Baby*, recognized this barrier. She was harsher in her analysis of these mothers than was Spock, for whom this feeling appeared normal. Pryor stated, "An occasional truly neurotic mother, breast feeding against her real wishes, cannot give herself to the baby at all. There are, after all, frigid breast feeders just as there are frigid wives. In such a case, the physical aspects of motherhood are a source of distress to both partners, and bottle feeding is gladly substituted."[26]

Neither Spock nor Pryor suggested any further exploration of these mothers' feelings or decisions. By contrast, Niles Newton reported that an aversion to breast feeding often accompanied a woman's dissatisfaction with her life situation or with that of women in general. Such dissatisfaction would seem to warrant further exploration rather than simply advising bottle feeding as the better choice.[27] As Spock himself pointed out, it was often a culturally influenced decision rather than one made based on full information about breast feeding.

A second aspect of medical advice contrasts with La Leche League tenets. Physicians regularly underestimated the superiority of breast milk. As the sense that the infant mortality crisis had been conquered became prevalent, physicians played down the nutritional and immunological advantages of breast milk. Like many of his predecessors, Spock held that breast milk was a superior infant food while simultaneously discounting the importance of this fact. Thus, his statement that breast feeding was natural and that, in general, it was safer to choose "the natural way unless you are absolutely sure you have a better way" was not forceful in itself and was further weakened by the general tenor of his breast-feeding advice. For instance, he was skeptical about the immunological properties of colostrum (the first fluid produced by the breast following birth). Therefore, he saw no problem in the hospital practice of often delaying the first nursing until twelve or more hours after birth.[28] The *Better Homes and Gardens Baby Book*, on the other hand, considered ingestion of the colostrum important to the baby's health and encouraged nursing shortly after birth. This good advice is weakened by the editors' statement that because "very little milk" was obtained in the first few days, boiled water was to be offered between nursings.[29]

In a third contrast to League philosophy, doctors tended to schedule breast feeding rigidly. Many hospital maternity wards were run no differently than surgical wards. Regulations, major and minor, and schedules ruled nursing procedures. Babies and their mothers were expected to conform to these protocols. Mothers were frequently counseled to limit the length of feedings at first and to strive from the beginning for a feeding schedule. Mencken believed that a baby need be nursed only once on the day of birth and three times on the second and third days and that by the fourth day the mother and baby would be ready for feedings at shorter intervals. He advised two-hour intervals, except for seven hours at night. Babies, he believed, had "bad habits" that caused them to cry at night, but if allowed to cry three nights in a row, the baby would "never cry again."[30]

League mothers often reported discouraging encounters with this rigidity. Such was the experience of Virginia Matson, of Waukegan, Illinois. When Matson was expecting her third baby, she was determined to nurse, although she had not succeeded in nursing her first two children. She was convinced that hospital routine had been the reason for her past problems. Her doctor confirmed this. "He explained that he felt that the best method of obtaining full nursing was to follow the time-honored technique of nursing the baby whenever the baby cried and not to follow any rigid time schedule." In spite of this advice, he also conceded that babies were brought out on a definite schedule and given complementary feedings as a practical way to solve hospital work problems.[31]

Both Spock's book and the *Better Homes and Gardens Baby Book* also insisted that for the first few nursings the nursing period should be limited. Spock suggested fifteen minutes. The *Better Homes and Gardens Baby Book* suggested that five minutes was long enough for each feeding for the first few days. These medical advisors also tightly regulated the frequency of nursings. Carefully regulated schedules were worked out with the ultimate goal of limiting feedings to every four hours during the day and eliminating night feedings as soon as possible. Feeding was limited to one breast, unless this practice left the baby unsatisfied. If the baby was still hungry, doctors suggested more frequent feedings and giving both breasts. The goal of these more frequent nursings, however, continued to be getting the baby to return to the four-hour schedule. Like adults in the increasingly technological workplace, infants were expected to live by a mechanical clock.

In a fourth contrast with League advice, when infants failed to gain weight on breast milk, physicians commonly relied on supplements rather than improved nursing technique to solve the problem. For Spock,

supplementing with formula if the baby was "miserably hungry or continues to lose weight" was the necessary choice. He believed that the
supplemental bottle, which he advised the mother to give after each
breast feeding, would be needed only temporarily in many cases. If this
breast-plus-bottle method did not increase the supply of breast milk,
however, Spock held that the mother might wean her baby to the bottle,
assured that she had tried as hard as she could. Spock's concern that mothers not become overly anxious about breast-feeding difficulties led him to
offer advice that would almost certainly assure the end of breast feeding.

The *Better Homes and Gardens Baby Book* took exception to this practice. Its editors wrote, "At the present time [1951], many young mothers
are being defeated in their efforts to nurse their babies because hospitals
and doctors are too quick to offer a formula as supplement to mother's
milk in the early stage of nursing and because babies are given bottles of
formula in the nursery to stop their crying."[32] Despite this awareness,
most hospitals continued to follow the same principles Spock advised.

In common with many other practitioners, Spock could see no harm
in adding supplementary feeding to breast feeding right from birth. In
fact, he not only saw no harm in this practice but perceived advantages to
giving *all* breast-fed babies a bottle at least twice a week. He reasoned
that the mother might become ill or have to go out of town in an
emergency. In such cases, the necessary weaning would be easier for a
baby who was already accustomed to a bottle. Behind this advice were
two assumptions: a mother's serious illness would necessitate weaning
the baby for the sake of her health and because of her possible hospital-
ization; and if the mother had to leave town, the baby would have to stay
behind because babies were not very portable. Thus, physicians recommended supplementary bottles not only to ameliorate nutritional problems but also to relieve mothers of a tied-down feeling. Such beliefs per-
sisted well past the midcentury. In 1988, Dr. Christopher Green wrote
that, in a time when shared parenting was becoming more valued, breast
feeding as an unshared activity played havoc with an equal division of
labor.[33] Indirectly these assumptions follow on an initial acceptance that
the advantages of breast feeding are insignificant, that science's own
invention, the infant formula, is as healthy as breast milk.

A fifth way common infant-feeding practices interfered with breast
feeding was through the introduction of solid foods before the infant
was six months old. Doctors believed that healthy babies could tolerate

strained foods in small amounts almost from birth, and though Spock noted that "a baby taking his first teaspoonful of solid food is quite funny and a little pathetic," he gave parents several suggestions for making the process eventually successful. While other pediatricians advised waiting considerably longer before introducing solids, many continued to counsel parents to follow rigid rules for the introduction of solids. Few were as relaxed about the feeding of solids as Green, who suggested, "First see what happens when the chosen food is put in his mouth. If it is sucked up with the whoosh of a vacuum cleaner, then you're probably on the right track."[34]

A sixth factor interfered with successful nursing. Even if no emergency weaning occurred and mothers themselves were contentedly breast feeding, physicians regularly recommended a combination of breast and bottle feeding because this made weaning to the bottle more gradual and easier on both baby and mother. Physicians assumed that the infant would be weaned to a bottle because most mothers would not want to nurse a baby for the full year necessary for optimum health. Spock advised that breast-fed infants be weaned from the breast by eight to twelve months. By that time, he believed, the nursing baby would be ready for a cup. Despite his acceptance of the fact that bottle-fed babies were often "unwilling to give up the bottle until they are well over a year old," he strongly believed that prolonging breast feeding was detrimental because "it is likely to become a habit that makes him unnaturally dependent on his mother."[35] While the *Better Homes and Gardens Baby Book* expressed no such concerns, its editors believed weaning should occur on a regulated week-to-week schedule so that "baby will be weaned without annoyance to anyone."[36] Smith believed that "the eruption of teeth is nature's way of telling the mother that solid foods are more important than milk."[37] It is interesting to note that Smith, the scientific expert, here calls on "nature" as his guide.

The seventh contrast between League philosophy and most approaches to child care is their different understandings of the father-infant relationship. Whereas mid-twentieth-century understandings of the father's role were less rigid than those of previous eras, they tended to equate an increased role for fathers with bottle feeding. Spock reflected the increasing interest in the father's role in infant care. He held it was wrong to think that the care of babies and children should be left entirely to the mother. Nevertheless, he equated "real fatherhood" with the bottle-fed infant. He saw opportunities for fathering in preparing formula on weekends and in feeding an infant its 2 A.M. bottle. The fact that a father could feed a bottle-fed baby was often used as a pro-bottle argument. Palmer noted that many men admitted they were jealous of the breast-feeding relationship between mother and child.[38]

Spock also considered the disinterestedness of some fathers as unimportant. "Of course, there are some fathers who would get goose flesh at the very idea of helping to take care of a baby, and there's no good to be gained from trying to force them."[39] In his chapter on breast feeding, there is no mention of the baby's father. The father was reintroduced into Spock's book 247 sections later, in a chapter entitled "Managing Young Children." Spock warned fathers against being overly impatient with their sons, because boys needed to feel comfortable with their fathers so they could pattern themselves after them. As for girls, Spock said it was not so easy to see what a girl needed from her father, yet girls needed their father's friendly approval so that they could feel confident in themselves. "I'm thinking of little things like approving of her dress, or hair-do, or the cookies she's made."[40]

Finally, and most important, the medical community engendered in women an enormous defeatism in the face of breast-feeding difficulties. In the 1950s, one mother, Helen Kreigh, wrote, "It seems almost as though the modern woman has accepted a defeatist attitude toward breast feeding. Too often she doesn't back up her body with her will. . . . In the hospital I heard a nurse ask a new mother if she were planning to breast-feed her baby. The reply was a hesitant, 'I want to if I can,' but the tone said, 'I know I'll fail.'" Kreigh remembered having similar feelings herself just after the birth of her first child. These fears, she was certain, were brought about by overly cautious advice that warned her to not feel discouraged if her baby should refuse to take the breast.[41]

It was difficult for mothers to challenge the defeatist attitude of a society in which breast feeding had ceased to be the norm and where bottle feeding was the acceptable way to handle any difficulties a mother might experience in nursing. In 1931, the editors of the *Journal of the American Medical Association* frankly admitted that breast feeding had become irksome if not actually difficult for many mothers of their time. Although they did not accept this as an argument against breast feeding, they offered it as a consolation because they saw the change in the mode of infant nutrition as a new imperative.[42]

Although most breast-feeding problems can be solved through education, some are quite complex. As La Leche League leader and mother of four Dorothy Brewster wrote, "Breastfeeding is not totally instinctive. Successful lactation is a confidence trick, and accomplishing it in difficult situations is best achieved with knowledge and emotional support."[43] When women turned to their doctors for help in solving these problems, they were more likely to be told to wean the baby to the bottle because doctors had little formal education in handling such problems and a great deal in directing formula feeding. Part of the problem was that breast feeding fell in a "medical no-man's-land." A woman's breasts were the concern of her obstetrician, who had no specialized training in infant feeding. Breast milk was the concern of the pediatrician. Thus, increasing the milk supply became the pediatrician's job. Prescribing medication to dry up the milk supply was done by an obstetrician. No matter whom a mother called, she stood a good chance of being hindered rather than helped by the doctor's advice.

Palmer noted that the same medical traditions that "destroy breast-feeding are sanctified by recommendations in textbooks and training schools." When she read through the pamphlets distributed by the British Health Service to mothers, she discovered an emphasis on the risks of inadequate breast milk running side by side with advertisements for artificial formula.[44] I discovered the same phenomenon in American popular literature directed at new mothers. Alongside most articles promoting breast feeding ran advertisements for formula, baby foods, cod liver oil, vitamins, and laxatives, all unnecessary for the healthy breast-fed infant.

The extension of the ideology of scientific motherhood to breast feeding meant that mothers wishing to nurse were given advice that, because garnered from facts about artificial feeding, often contributed to the failure of the attempt to breast-feed. Between World War I and the 1950s, although physicians and child-care educators continued to recommend breast milk as the best infant food, more and more advice on infant feeding began with a nod to the advantages and benefits of nursing and then discussed bottle feeding in great detail. La Leche League reversed this trend by offering an alternative approach. For La Leche League, women, not the doctors, were the "experts" when it came to infant feeding and child care.

chapter 3

. . . .

An Alternative Approach
Maternal Knowing

CORRECT INFORMATION WITHIN
A SUPPORTIVE NETWORK

La Leche League did not altogether reject the ideology of scientific motherhood. Its manual was not intended as a substitute for valuable medical research. The founders were familiar with many books, pamphlets, and articles written by doctors and nurses. They quoted these sources frequently and recommended many of them as reading for new mothers.

The League sought to correct scientific misinformation by directing mothers to the most adequate and supportive scientific information. Mary White had suffered through inadequate information. With her first three infants, she quickly succumbed to bottles for three reasons: one, her baby was drowsy from medication she was given during childbirth; two, she was informed on the first day that she did not have enough milk and supplements were necessary; and three, she and her baby went home to a mother-oriented, bottle-feeding schedule. Several of the founders had similar experiences. Therefore, the League's clearest self-perception

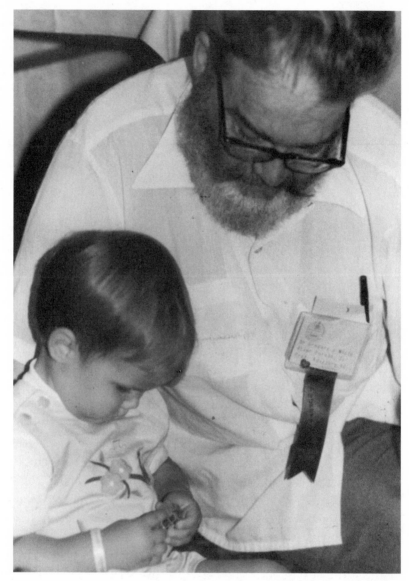

Dr. Gregory White has been a medical advisor for La Leche League since its beginning as well as the family doctor for many of its earliest members. Here he sits quietly entertaining a toddler while listening to a speaker at La Leche League's twenty-fifth-anniversary conference.

was that it served as a conduit of correct information within a supportive network. It offered alternative approaches to replace misinformation about breast feeding, which it perceived as potentially troublesome to successful nursing.

BREAST-FED IS BEST FED

Doctors often underemphasized the importance of breast feeding, even when they admitted that it was the best method of infant feeding. The League took strong exception to this attitude. "Mothering through breastfeeding is the most natural and effective way of understanding and satisfying the needs of the baby."[1] Why, League mothers asked, should a mother who nourished her baby completely for nine months in the womb suddenly entertain doubts about her continuing ability to nurture her newborn? Because, the League suggested, the medical profession, in its role of assisting nature, developed a substitute formula for the rare baby who could not get breast milk. While this worked, it was still only a substitute, something better than nothing in the exceptional case. Yet, somehow the exception became the rule.

The League's goal was to render bottle feeding once again the exception. One way of accomplishing this, League members believed, was to educate mothers who had already expressed an interest in breast feeding, to help them believe they were making a choice that would benefit themselves and their infants. For the League, the physical and psychological benefits of breast feeding accrued to both mother and infant.

In its earliest edition of *The Womanly Art of Breastfeeding*, the League stressed two major physical benefits for mothers: less blood loss after birth and natural spacing of children. As to the psychological benefits, the manual quoted several physicians who promoted breast feeding as a way to build motherly love and to foster a feeling of motherly confidence. Breast feeding was a way to continue the intimacy of pregnancy. And as Karen Pryor's *Nursing Your Baby* pointed out, "The mother, like the baby, needs to be shown that she is loved; and the behavior of even a tiny baby at the breast is proof positive of that."[2]

Proponents of bottle feeding often emphasized that mothers *need* a break from their babies so as not to become fatigued. The League claimed that nursing was "nature's way" of helping mothers relax and rest. The nursing mother has a compelling reason for taking necessary, healthy, and reviving breaks at regular intervals during the day. League literature urged mothers to avoid fatigue so as to maintain a good let-down reflex. Breast feeding became in League philosophy not something a mother needed a break from but the very source of her breaks from the myriad of other demands on her time and energy.

Gabrielle Palmer enumerated some additional physical benefits to the mother. The breast-feeding hormone prolactin augments the rate at which vitamin D is converted to its active form; this, in turn, enhances calcium utilization. Further, women who breast-fed were less likely to develop breast cancer. She noted, "The topic is rarely discussed publicly, perhaps with the worthy but mistaken and dangerous motive of protecting women's feelings. Women have the right to know about their own bodies."[3]

La Leche League was more cautious on this subject. The 1981 edition of *The Womanly Art of Breastfeeding* stated that the question of whether breast feeding helped protect a woman from breast cancer was still being studied. "The search is complicated by the fact that other factors, can, and probably do, influence the rate of cancer in a population." The League did not, however, altogether discount this possible benefit. The League did not wish to set aside this important consideration, but also, consistent with its own incorporation of an altered "scientific motherhood," it was not about to rush in with unsubstantiated claims.

According to La Leche League belief, babies, as well as mothers, benefited enormously from breast feeding. When the League began, many pediatricians demonstrated a laissez-faire attitude about the possible psychological benefits of breast feeding for the baby. In contrast, the League stressed such advantages. The League unequivocally stated, "The baby has a basic need for his mother's love and presence which is as intense as his need for food. This need remains even though his mother may be absent for a period of time for needs or reasons of her own."[4] From the beginning this was a strong League conviction. As the League grew, it offered scientific studies that supported the idea that mothers who breast-fed tended to interact with their infants with different behaviors from bottle-feeding mothers. These behaviors included more frequent feedings and longer feeding durations and more touching, cuddling, and rocking of the infant at nonfeeding times. These studies advanced the notion that this increased contact deepened the psychosocial relationship between the breast-feeding mother and her infant. La Leche League held that such differences could have a long-term effect on the child's development. The intimacy developed during infancy would help a mother remain closely attuned to her baby as he or she moved into the busyness of the toddler years, a prime time for learning.

The League wished to remain nonjudgmental of bottle-feeding mothers without diluting the impact of its message to women who wished to breast-feed. League mothers knew that bottle-feeding mothers and babies loved each other, yet they were convinced that happy nursing couples felt different about each other. They themselves had found that they were poignantly aware of having different feelings when they had bottle-fed one or two children and then breast-fed subsequent babies. The physical intimacy of breast feeding eroded the barriers that exist between individuals in a way that no amount of conscientious mothering could do. This rapport continued to be a part of their relationship with their child long after weaning.

THE SUPERIOR INFANT FOOD

"Breast milk is the superior infant food," League members proclaimed from the beginning. They never accepted the common medical opinion that a well-chosen and correctly prepared formula could be so close to breast milk that the differences between the two were not a prime factor for a mother deciding between breast and bottle feeding. League material has always underscored two main reasons bottle feeding remains a second best to breast feeding: breast milk is nutritionally superior to even the best of formulas, and the immunological benefits of breast milk are both far-reaching and inimitable.

The League insisted on several ways in which breast milk is a superior infant food. First, breast milk is specifically designed by "Nature" for human babies; it is easier to digest, thus conserving the baby's energy for better physical and neurological growth. The League pointed out past medical failures to recognize that breast milk contains certain elements that, when left out of formulas, had caused babies to become seriously ill or even die. In the first edition of its manual, the League recognized that contemporary formulas were much improved over earlier versions. Nevertheless, the founders were still concerned. There remained unknown components in human milk. This rendered any substitute, even if composed of elements currently known to be needed, perhaps lacking in some equally essential factor not yet discovered in human milk. A lack of any one of the components could be a serious disadvantage to the baby.

The 1963 edition of the manual reiterated the faith in the superiority of breast milk expressed in the original. It made one new point that clearly reflected the later era: "Another consideration of some importance in this atomic age is the presence in milk of such products of radioactive fallout as strontium-90. . . . The consensus of scientific thought is that the amount of such radiation-emitting bodies present in breast milk is significantly smaller than that found in formula milk."[5]

By 1981, increasing research and an expanded format for the manual allowed the League to devote an entire chapter to the superiority of breast milk. The chapter contrasted the many differences between cow's milk and mother's milk. It explored the composition of both in detail, discussing proteins, fats, lactose, vitamins, and minerals. It demonstrated that two supplements, vitamin D and iron, often advised for breast-fed babies, are not necessary. In the past, research had shown breast milk to be low in iron and deficient in vitamin D. More recent studies revealed that the amount of iron in breast milk was ideal for the human infant and that additional iron could be dangerous. Other studies showed that previous researchers had been looking for vitamin D in the curd rather than the whey of the breast milk. The League also noted the new research on contaminants in breast milk. Some physicians were responding to this research by advising mothers to avoid nursing. The manual suggested that this was a radical approach that unnecessarily deprived the baby of the many benefits of breast feeding. Rather, the authors suggested, "By giving some serious thought to what you eat and the products you use in your home, you can help sweep your immediate environment clean and thus lower the amount of contamination you, your baby, and the rest of the family receive."[6]

Second, the League held that allergies are more common in artificially fed babies than in those who nursed. These allergies, begun in infancy, might continue for many years. Allergic reactions to artificial food can be so severe that they actually threaten the life of a baby. It was ironic, the second edition of *The Womanly Art of Breastfeeding* noted, that because formula feeding had become the standard feeding method, mothers might actually be heard to remark, "sometimes rather proudly, 'Such-and-such didn't agree with Johnny; the doctor had to prescribe *three* (or maybe *four*, or even *five*) different formulas before he found one that agreed with him.' Meanwhile, poor Johnny!"[7]

Third, breast-fed babies were healthier. The League called breast milk "nature's vaccine," a name the founders learned from Dr. Herbert Ratner. Research, they discovered, supported their own conviction. The baby was born with a supply of antibodies received via the placenta. They were manufactured by the mother's immune system in response to infections the mother had been exposed to. These included the common contagious diseases of childhood. Although the mother's immunity to these diseases lasted for her lifetime, the protection passed to her unborn child was temporary. Therefore, the antibodies that were present in breast milk were important to prolong this natural immunity. Colostrum, the fluid that proceeds the milk and continues to be present in diminishing amounts in breast milk, contains protective white blood cells — leukocytes — the body's chief defense against infections. The concentration of leukocytes in breast milk is about the same as in blood.[8]

Before they were even aware of this research, the mothers of La Leche League had noticed that when they fed their babies entirely on breast milk, the babies did not get constipated, were less likely to develop other serious digestive upsets, and caught fewer serious respiratory infections than did formula-fed babies.[9] In the first edition of the manual, the founders claimed, "Breast feeding definitely prolongs the period of natural immunity to virus diseases." They recognized that the study they quoted was done before the discovery of penicillin but still held that prevention is better than cure. The second edition repeated this basic information, adding that for the premature infant, breast milk is especially important because of colostrum's disease-fighting properties. Colostrum contains five or six times as much protein as the later milk and only half as much fat and carbohydrates, which are not as easily digested by the newborn baby. In other words, the League claimed that no formula could ever be *better* than breast milk. And no matter how nearly science was able to approximate breast milk, the importance of breast feeding in the mother-child relationship would remain.

Better dental health and facial formation was a fourth claim the League manuals made in support of breast-feeding babies. Researchers discovered that the easier sucking that bottle nipples afforded was bad for babies. The long, hard artificial nipple used in bottle feeding could promote underdeveloped facial structure while a mother's nipple enhanced facial development, thus preparing the baby's tongue and mouth to make the complex adjustments needed to form the sounds needed to speak clearly.

In support of these claims, the League pointed to several studies done in New Zealand in the 1970s. Discoveries such as these prompted Gerber to develop the NUK Orthodontic Nipple and the NUK Orthodontic Pacifier-Exerciser. These replaced the old hard nipples and were designed to resemble a nursing mother's nipple so that, like a mother's breast, they encouraged oral exercise. La Leche League recognized the superiority of the NUK nipple over previous models. League leaders might recommend it in emergency situations that called for the temporary use of a bottle; however, the temporariness of such situations was always emphasized.

BREAST FEEDING, THE
BEST EMOTIONAL BEGINNING

League mothers were convinced that science, as well as experience, verified that breast milk was the superior infant food. Yet League mothers continued to accent the mother-child relationship as the most important benefit of breast feeding. This was a vulnerable point in their ideology because the empirical findings about the biological specificity of breast milk were more readily verified than were claims about emotional benefits such as increased security. The needs of individual humans within a specific cultural context present a complex array of factors that make it difficult to make solidly unquestionable claims about the emotional benefits of one way of infant feeding over another.

The League, however, placed full faith in its claim that a baby's emotional needs are just as strong, just as important, as his or her physical needs. League mothers understood a baby's need for his or her mother's closeness, for cuddling in her arms, to be as urgent as his or her need to be fed and kept warm and dry. The League recognized that all an infant's emotional needs would not be met by breast feeding alone. League mothers, however, held that the breast-feeding mother was more likely than was the bottle-feeding mother to develop the sensitive attentiveness that would enable her to tell whether a baby was crying out of hunger, tiredness, frustration, pain, or discomfort.

La Leche League insisted that the sooner the baby was put to the breast the better. "The sucking reflex of a full-term healthy newborn was usually at peak about twenty to thirty minutes after he was born, provided he was not drowsy from drugs or anesthesia used during labor and delivery." Early breast feeding also benefited the mother by hastening the delivery of the placenta. In home births, nursing without delay after birth helped the mother and baby to get off to a good start, thus posing fewer breast-feeding problems. On the other hand, hospital deliveries were another situation. Mothers might not be allowed to nurse for twelve to twenty-four hours because of various complications of medicated deliveries. These included problems with hospital practices such as routinely putting all newborns under an overhead heat lamp, "a procedure that is rarely necessary," but League leaders reassured mothers that if the first nursings were delayed or did not go well, gradually, as they had more quiet times together, "the magical wand of mother love imperceptibly brushes over, and strong bonds are formed between mother and child."[10]

In the 1970s, this concept of mother-infant bonding became a major concern of infant research. Dr. Marshall Klaus's book, *Maternal-Infant Bonding*, was widely read. The League held that artificial schedules suppressed and distorted attachment behavior, whereas a baby-led schedule promoted bonding:

Thus mothers shape their babies' choices and dispositions. So, mothers, if you want a smiley baby, respond *before* the crying starts. If you tend to wait for crying, you will have a baby that tends to cry.

When things are going smoothly, we may see no evidence of attachment behavior. Mothers and babies may appear to be indifferent to each other. Only let some threat appear and you will see it at once, because attachment behavior exists for the purpose of insuring proximity between mother and baby so that babies will be safe and cared for.[11]

However, the League warned leaders to be careful of their use of the term "bonding" because some seemed to have "picked up the notion that mother-baby bonding takes place during the first hour or so following birth, and after that, nevermore!" Rather, Klaus held that humans have a tremendous capacity for "adaptation, learning, change." Although the very early hours after birth might be an especially sensitive period, it was not a critical one for humans. "But anywhere along the line, however unpropitious the beginning, change is possible, in the marvelously complex human baby—or human adult."[12]

FORGET THE CLOCK, ENJOY THE BABY

The League also took a relaxed attitude toward the amount of milk that an infant received. The first edition of the manual emphasized that a mother could not know in ounces how much the baby received from her. This is a point that the League would continue to reiterate. It was not necessary, League leaders insisted, to know this. They advised against the weighing in and out after each feeding that many doctors suggested because it was unnecessary and a nuisance that would be sure to cause the mother anxiety. Better indications that the baby is receiving enough milk are whether he or she is content, has good bowel movements, and wets fairly often.

As to the four-hour schedule, the manual claimed a baby was doing very well indeed if he or she went four or more hours between feedings even once a day. At the heart of the League's approach is its belief that there are no rules, that each mother-baby combination is different, and that each mother and child needs to become acquainted in their own way. Mothers, not doctors, are the true experts on infant care. Newborn infants usually nurse every two to three hours, even occasionally needing to nurse every hour to build up milk supply. This includes nights. To ensure a well-rested mother, another prerequisite of a good milk supply, the League recommends that when an infant wakes at night, the mother tuck him into bed with her, start nursing him, and the two of them can drop off to sleep together. League mothers reassured new mothers that this procedure was quite safe and that they had all done it. Such advice was a far cry from the *Better Homes and Gardens Baby Book*'s suggestion that "a room of Baby's own should go to the top of your list" when parents were preparing for the arrival of their infant.[13]

Also in contrast to common medical advice, the League did not recommend limiting the amount of time the baby spent at the breast, because it could lead to understimulation and a reduction in milk supply. League mothers suggested giving both breasts at each feeding, especially in the early weeks of nursing, and allowing the baby to remain at the second breast for at least twenty minutes and longer if both mother and baby were content.

The League faced another significant challenge. Breast-feeding mothers' expectations were highly influenced by the bottle-feeding culture that surrounded them. The frequent feedings a breast-fed baby initially required could make a mother experience her infant as insatiable, because she had heard so much about the four-hour schedule. Pryor reminded mothers that a breast-fed baby would most likely be three months old before he or she could go three hours between feedings. It was not surprising, therefore, that so many mothers could not nurse their babies when a four-hour schedule was so often insisted on from birth and when it was also customary to advise mothers to nurse from one breast only at each feeding. "The woman who secreted so much milk that she could feed a baby adequately, despite the limited sucking stimulation given by offering only one breast every four hours, must have been rare indeed."[14]

The League viewed its no-schedule approach as logical since it held that "a baby's wants are a baby's needs." Feeding a baby according to his own time schedule was a major component of meeting his needs. The manual stressed that a concern with how often a baby nurses was a modern Western focus. League literature frequently carried narratives to illustrate that this was never an issue for mothers living in cultures that were less characterized by mechanization and rigid schedules. In these societies, a mother "doesn't need to count how often she feeds the baby any more than she counts how often she kisses the baby."[15]

In 1988 Palmer found that restricting the time a baby spent at the breast was still standard medical practice in the West. Doctors and nurses often believed, she noted, that nursing could cause sore nipples. In fact, it was not sucking that damaged nipples. Rather, it was bad positioning of the baby and frequent washing that were the culprits. These medical rules, based on misinformation, could sabotage the baby's natural way of maintaining a sufficient milk supply for his individual needs.[16]

The League offered mothers many ways of dealing with sore nipples that did not interfere with this natural process. It warned mothers to use only clear water to wash their nipples after each feeding because soap was drying and could lead to cracked nipples. Breast milk itself acts as an antiseptic agent on nipple skin. Also, shortening nursing to overcome sore nipples actually made the problem worse. Longer nursings were easier on the breast because they prevented engorgement and toughened the nipples. Applying ice for a few minutes before and after nursing was suggested to ease any discomfort. Because the League recognized that these simple measures might not suffice for some mothers, it offered additional informational pamphlets on sore nipples and actually devoted several pages of the third edition of the manual to this problem. This approach typified the League attitude that Western culture treated the successful breast-feeding mother like a rarity when just the opposite was the truth. Most mothers could breast-feed if given the correct information.

The League encouraged the medical world to adopt this viewpoint. Jan Riordan's *A Practical Guide to Breastfeeding* was directed at nurses and included detailed instructions on how a nurse could be certain that an infant was properly positioned for nursing and latched on correctly, both of which were important to avoid sore nipples. She suggested the short-term use of a NUK pacifier as a way to help a baby correct a faulty sucking pattern.[17] The League itself was cautious about the use of pacifiers. The manual suggested that if a baby had nursed shortly before but howled, chewed its fist, or sucked on anything available, the mother might want to consider a pacifier. But she ought to continue to hold the baby until he settled down. The League, always wary of any substitute for breast feeding, warned that in using a pacifier, a parent might pacify a symptom but not relieve the cause.

HOLDING OFF ON SUPPLEMENTS: THE "NATURAL" APPROACH

"For the healthy, full-term baby breast milk is the only food necessary until baby shows signs of needing solids, about the middle of the first year of life."[18] This statement was the fourth in what La Leche League called its "ten basic concepts." The League considered this concept vital to successful breast feeding. When this practice was not followed, especially in the first eight weeks, League mothers believed, failure at breast feeding was a likely result.

Because they so firmly believed that supplements sabotage the breast-feeding process, the founders and all subsequent leaders warned mothers wishing to breast-feed to be prepared to assert themselves on this issue. Hospital routines in the mid-twentieth century and successful breast feeding were at odds, so the League recommended that mothers be certain that their doctors fully understood that supplementary formula is one of the biggest deterrents to establishing a good milk supply. They were also advised to request that their doctors leave firm orders with the hospital staff forbidding supplements, formula, or water and asking that the baby be brought to the mother when he was hungry. The manual told mothers to remind nurses and doctors frequently that they were determined to nurse and did not want stilbestrol, the "drying-up" pills that were sometimes routinely given. Leaders also warned against taking formula home. If it were not in the house, a mother would be less tempted to use it in a moment of doubt.

Slow weight gain, one of the factors often cited by physicians as a reason for supplementing breast feeding, was rarely considered by League mothers as a reason to discontinue nursing. Rather, League leaders and the physicians who supported them suggested several other approaches. First, slow weight gain might not be a problem in some situations. Although the founders suggested that a pound a month is a good gain, they warned mothers whose babies gained less not to conclude immediately that they did not have enough milk. In some families, it was the normal pattern. Dorothy Brewster related this story: "One mother who had been told to wean each of her first four babies because of their slow weight gain was determined she would breastfeed her fifth. When the suggestion again came to wean, she was prepared with growth charts from the first four babies showing that even on formula her babies were just slow gainers."[19]

In situations where the mother and the doctor had determined that slow weight gain was not simply this baby's pattern, the League suggested solutions that did not rely on supplementing breast feeding. Mothers could offer the breast more frequently. In addition, to properly empty the breast and stimulate the milk supply the infant must be grasping the whole aureola (pinkish area around the nipples). League literature contained many suggestions on how to encourage this sucking pattern. In another aspect of establishing good breast-feeding patterns, the baby often labeled as "such a good baby" because he regularly slept for four- and five-hour intervals might actually be too placid for his own best health. If such a baby was gaining weight at less than the optimum, he might need a reversal of "demand feeding." In other words, the mother might need to wake him every two hours and encourage him to nurse until his weight gain stabilized. Also, if the infant tended to fall asleep before nursing on both breasts, diaper changing or some other quiet activity at midfeeding might rouse the baby so he could give the breasts adequate stimulation.

Finally, if a mother was overly anxious either about her ability to breast-feed or about some other life situation, this could interfere with her let-down, or milk-ejection, reflex and inhibit lactation. The League sought to give the mother the confidence she needed and encouraged her to make her own situation as calm and happy as possible. For this reason, League leaders discouraged the practice of weighing in and out after each feed-ing, which, they believed, was certain to make the whole process more anxiety causing. In fact, League mothers often offered sitting down for a nursing as the best way to become less anxious and calmer in crisis situa-tions.[20] One confidence drainer was comparing the size of one's own baby to that of another baby of the same age. Advertisements for formula inevitably pictured chubby babies to promote the products. The exam-ples were numerous, but one particularly ill-informed advertisement ap-peared in *Good Housekeeping* in 1907. It pictured twins, a girl, breast-fed from birth, and a boy, "raised on Mellin's food." The little girl, while quite healthy appearing, was considerably smaller than her brother. The adver-tisement read, "This ought to convince you of the great merits of Mellin food." Later, the text added, "We do not claim that Mellin's food and milk is better than mother's milk." Yet the contrast between breast-fed and Mellin-fed was at the heart of the claim for Mellin as the best artificial formula "in the world." Thus, nursing mothers worried when their in-fants were not as heavy as some formula-fed infants.

One breast-feeding mother related to her doctor that her baby's grand-mother was concerned that he was gaining weight too slowly and urged the mother to give him a bottle of juice or some cereal. The doctor answered, "Your baby is doing fine; he's a very healthy baby. He is small but every baby is a different person." Not all doctors were as reassuring. Another mother reported that her doctor showed considerable alarm at her baby's slow weight gain, and it took the knowledge she had gained at La Leche League meetings to convince the doctor that the baby need not be put on supplements.

League mothers also faced the accusation that a breast-fed baby who was plump was gaining too much. In defense, the League noted that Dr. Derrick Jelliffe held that the exclusively breast-fed baby might appear to be overweight but was not ever obese. Therefore, the League warned mothers against allowing their babies to be "put on a diet." Heredity, it held, was a defining factor in the larger baby's size just as it was for the smaller-than-average infant. Rather than become overly concerned about a baby's chubbiness, the League suggested that mothers ask themselves whether their babies were happy and alert. The manual reminds mothers that "fat accumulated in the relatively inactive pre-toddler stage is preparatory for the highly active time when the busy toddler hardly has time to eat."[21]

La Leche League also resisted the twentieth-century trend to an earlier introduction of solids. From the beginning, the League insisted that around six months was the best time to offer a baby's first solids. Following this plan assured the maintenance of a good milk supply. If solids are introduced when the baby is around two months old, breast milk may dry up by the time he or she is five or six months old.

From their own observations, League mothers noted several other problems that could arise from introducing solids too early. Introducing solids before a baby was ready could begin a struggle over food between parents and baby. This could lead to similar problems throughout the child's life and even contribute to eating disorders later. In terms of physiological development, before six months the baby's immature digestive system had difficulty utilizing solid foods without upsets, so introducing solids could actually be harmful. Finally, many foods that later might cause no problems generated allergies when introduced too soon.

Pryor added that the younger a baby was when solids were introduced the sooner the mother's menses would return. Because many League mothers were interested in natural birth control, the delay in ovulation that often accompanied the delay in menstruation was important. Just the same, the League developed its policy on the introduction of solid foods around concerns about the baby's health, growth, and development rather than around the attempt to prevent ovulation. This latter benefit was the less certain of the two because suppression of ovulation was influenced by many factors.[22]

HOW LONG DO THOSE LA LECHE LEAGUE BABIES NURSE?

Mary White recalled asking her husband when their first child was six weeks old, "How long am I going to be nursing this baby?" When he replied that it would probably be six months, she was horrified. White was most likely the first in a long line of mothers "horrified" when they first heard La Leche League's weaning policy: "Ideally, the breastfeeding relationship will continue until the baby outgrows the need."[23] This was perhaps the most controversial aspect of the League's ideology and the one that turned many mothers away. Certain convictions stood behind it.

The key to the League's weaning policy was the belief that a mother could surely rely on her own motherly instincts to know when her baby was ready for weaning. For La Leche League, motherly instincts were skills developed over the course of a caring, interactive relationship between mother and infant. Each set of "instincts" was individualized to meet the needs of a particular mother and infant. The League set some guidelines but urged mothers to have faith that they knew their own babies best. The founders, even while advising a procedure that contrasted strongly to that of most baby "experts" of their day, still maintained that it was not the League's purpose to work out a feeding schedule for any individual baby. This was a remarkable disclaimer considering that League guidelines include baby-led weaning, weaning gradually to the cup without an interim bottle-feeding period, and the expectation that weaning would be a slow process that might proceed well beyond a baby's first birthday. In the first edition of the manual, League leaders assured mothers, "Generally, breast fed babies are through nursing long before the bottle fed babies have given up the bottle — or their thumb."[24]

When the second edition of the manual came out, the founders faced societal expectations about weaning and the breast-fed baby in a more assertive manner than in the first edition. They pointed out that "a newborn at the breast is sometimes accepted in our American culture; an older baby, a toddler — never." Yet, in this same culture, "it is a common sight to see a two- or three-year-old with a bottle." They asked mothers to explore weaning the breast-fed baby as an issue separate from practices that concern bottle-fed babies. Breast feeding, they emphasized, was more than a means of assuring a baby superior nutrition. It was a relationship built around mutual needs, including comfort and affection as well as nourishment. Were nourishment the only goal, the authors asserted, it might be possible to bring nursing to an end earlier. "But if we view the nursing experience as a whole, if we see this important, intimate relationship as a vital part of motherhood, meeting the total psychosomatic needs of the baby, then it is hard to understand why we should set a specific time when this relationship *must* end."[25]

The League recognized that many physicians opposed this approach. Always careful to maintain a "scientific" base, however, the organization emphasized that many doctors, psychologists, and social anthropologists supported baby-led weaning. These scientists, the manual stated, "point out that in cultures where children are allowed to continue nursing quite freely as long as they like, the children in general are well-adjusted, gentle, agreeable persons when they grow up." League mothers found that, contrary to warnings that prolonged nursing would produce an overly dependent child, their toddlers who experienced the security of moving at their own pace actually traveled a very fast road to independence.[26]

As the League grew, individual mothers and their children modeled examples of baby-led weaning. The *La Leche League News* published narratives about a variety of weaning experiences. One mother wrote, "Every so often, I come across an article about a mother who wished her toddler would be willing to give up nursing. How I envy those mothers! My eleven-month-old son Nathaniel surprised me when he weaned himself at the tender age of eight months."[27]

Twyalia Voyles told a very different story. At the age of ten months, her daughter Alicia was nursing frequently. Thinking perhaps that she was nursing Alicia for every little thing just because that was the easiest way out, Twyalia decided that she would not offer Alicia the breast but also would not refuse it. The baby cut back for a while and then suddenly started wanting to nurse more when she became ill. During that period, she would not eat any solids, so all she had was her mother's milk. Twyalia was grateful that her "mothering instincts" kept her from totally weaning because, if she had weaned the baby completely, she would not have had anything to really comfort her.[28]

Nursing an older baby or a toddler in a society that found this practice unacceptable remained a problem for many League members, despite their leaders' reassurances. Hearing and reading that prolonged breast feeding was perfectly natural and very beneficial to the baby still left mothers asking, "But when will he wean?" Dr. James Good offered this assurance: "There is no way a mother can force a child to nurse beyond the time he wishes." He also observed that no research had ever indicated that extended breast feeding caused psychological harm.

Rather, he warned against an overly early interruption of the mother-child relationship.[29]

Have faith in your child, League leaders urged. Realize that a nursing baby might seem to require a great deal of time and attention but, "before you know it, your baby is an active toddler, then in school, and your relationship as a nursing couple will be only a memory."[30]

THE MANLY ART OF FATHERING

From its inception, La Leche League has stressed the important contribution husbands and fathers make to successful breast feeding. League literature has always been written from the perspective of a household consisting of husband, wife, and child or children. The founders and their followers are convinced breast feeding and good mothering progress more easily in such an environment. They strongly believe children "naturally" flourish under the loving care of both a mother and a father. They also know this picture does not always hold true in real life and maintain that the satisfactions of nursing are available for every mother whatever her life situation. Still, almost all the family models presented in their literature are intact families with a mother and a father.

It is difficult today to realize how countercultural the League perspective on fatherhood was when compared to that of advisors such as Spock, who did not much concern themselves with the father's role in the early weeks of the baby's life.

Fathers were never pushed to the periphery of League philosophy but were understood from the beginning to be central figures in domestic life. The League expected a father to be his wife's mainstay during pregnancy, her comfort during childbirth, and very much in the foreground of child care. According to League philosophy, because the mother must care for the baby, the father must care for both the mother and baby. "Far from feeling shut out, he must realize that he is needed now as never before."[31]

Every edition of the manual contained a full chapter on fathering. Every fourth issue of the newsletter was devoted to stories about individual fathers. This literature outlined several aspects of the fathering role. First, a father's conviction that his baby had the *right* to his mother's milk could give his wife confidence. When the mother of a baby who always seemed hungry was about to run for a bottle, the father could

steady her, reminding her that babies cry for many reasons. League leaders suggested that the father fix his wife a snack and encourage her to call
an experienced breast-feeding mother. Also, he could stand between her
and those who would undermine her confidence, even when these de-
tractors included his mother or her own. Spock's book on child care
contained a longer section on selecting help for the new mother than on
the father's role in the care of his infant. In contrast, the League held that
when both parents had a clear understanding of the needs of family
members and the best way to meet those needs, the nuclear family was
capable of caring for itself.

Second, he could let his wife know that breast feeding enhanced her in
his eyes rather than making her less desirable, as some medical experts
suggested. This did not mean fathers would not feel jealous but only that
they would overcome these feelings as their own bond with the infant
grew. Sometimes, the mother had to be the one who reassured the father.
One young father wrote to Edwina Froehlich that he went through
some real suffering after his first baby was born. It seemed to him as
though all his wife's attention had been transferred from him to the baby.
It was his wife's continual reassurances that her love for him had inten-
sified, not diminished, that helped him through that hard time. One day
at a League get-together, he was talking with some other fathers and
discovered that his feelings had not been at all unusual.[32]

Third, a husband could assure his wife that while nursing she need not
"do all things well," that her well-being and the health of his children were
"greater values" than an immaculate home and intense community involvement. Rebecca Spradin certainly understood what such reassurance
could mean. She wrote that her husband Michael was the one who helped
her understand that all the projects she had planned because everyone had
told her that "all little babies do is eat and sleep" could be postponed until
her baby Aaron's needs for frequent nursing diminished.[33]

Finally, the League stressed that couples must give up old stereotypes
about who did what in the domestic circle. When children were young,
the founders wrote, time taking care of a fussy, ill, or needful infant
might leave a mother little time or energy for doing anything else. While
the manual did state that "there is, *on the whole*, a natural division of labor
within the family," it also claimed that fathers must not get trapped into
definitions of masculinity that would preclude them from taking an active role with their infants.[34] One father noted that because the gradual

easing into parenthood that a mother experienced through the physical and hormonal changes during pregnancy was denied to a father, he must work harder to adjust to parenthood. But, he wrote, "Although men have to work a little harder to adjust to parenthood, there may be a hidden advantage to this extra effort. Things you must work for are usually appreciated more."[35]

A COMPLEX PERSPECTIVE

La Leche League's perspective on fatherhood and the family, like the other aspects of its challenge to the traditional community of medical and psychological "experts," is a complex interweaving of the traditional, the chauvinist, and the countercultural. The League has been attacked by feminists for holding women to a stifling one-dimensional role. Yet many of the League's concepts liberated women from former limitations on their influence and their place—both in the family and in society. Although League philosophy widened the father's role within the family, the League also promoted gender roles that are often considered oppressive. Concerning a husband's role as companion, the second edition of the manual said, "A woman who has been in the house with small children all day needs adult companionship, especially that of her husband. She likes to hear what is going on 'in the world.'"[36]

Niles Newton presented a very different picture of La Leche League mothers. The League, she noted, attracted to its ranks extremely able and ethically sensitive women who, in a society that had devalued motherhood, focused first on their own families and at the same time woke "the industrial world to a value almost lost: the closeness of the breastfeeding mother-baby couple."[37] In her *Sex, Gender, and Christian Ethics*, Lisa Cahill stated that there are certain shared experiences that can form the foundation for social ethics. She noted that the most distinctively human of these are practical reason and affiliation with other human beings. "Positive human functioning in these areas is valued cross-culturally, and grounds morality."[38] La Leche League believed in the "shared experience" of breast feeding as one that can be valued cross-culturally.

chapter 4

. . . .

Feminism and
the Motherhood Wars

La Leche League promotes many tenets that many would consider non-feminist. League mothers center many life decisions around the needs of their infants. They make choices about employment that are popularly understood as sacrificing their own autonomy. Their ideal of shared parenthood rests on the concept of complementarity rather than strict equalitarianism. The organization itself has purposely chosen to remain outside many of the discussions at the heart of the women's movement. In spite of all these characteristics, though, League mothers are feminists. Their sense of self and their engagement with the world contrast sharply with the way most of their mothers lived their lives. And while many changes in contemporary culture account for these differences, the more subtle influences of the women's movement are among the most potent of these changes. To understand the relationship between League ideology and feminism, it is necessary to realize that feminism is neither a single impulse nor a newborn child of the late twentieth century.

Despite popular perceptions, women's roles have never been static, and especially from the advent of the Industrial Revolution through the

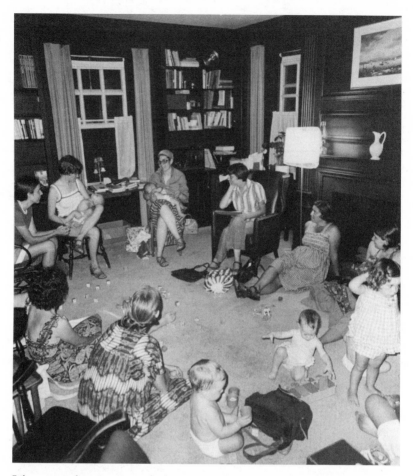

Like many other women in the late twentieth century, the members of La Leche League grow and gain strength through networking with other women. As in this photo, they gather in each other's homes to share parenting information and learn advocacy skills while their infants and toddlers play about them.

present day women's roles have evolved at an increasingly rapid pace. The earliest of these changes produced a society divided between what was considered public and what was viewed as private. The ideology of this division relegated women to the private sphere. Yet the reality of women's lives and of their aspirations conflicted with this ideology. By the mid-twentieth century, this resulted in an intense inquiry into the cultural values concerned with gender identity.

In the League's formative years fundamental questions about women's roles surfaced in an unprecedented manner. A "second wave" of feminism responded to these questions with a revolutionary understanding of women's place in society.[1] La Leche League's development of its basic concepts and the organization's approach to mothers were influenced by these changes in women's sense of self and their sense of community. Because the League focused on women's many roles, the League and feminism have over the last three decades confronted many of the same issues.

Furthermore, the two movements' ways of grounding their values in the religious dimension are similar. First, in both movements the religious influence is positive, though indirect. Second, both place a high value on grounding women's lives in networking for the common good. Despite these striking similarities, there are glaring differences as well.

As I place La Leche League within a cultural context that includes both feminist and conservative notions of women's roles in society, it becomes apparent that both currents of thought are important aspects of La Leche League philosophy. Neither a conservative traditional philosophy nor a feminist one can fully explicate La Leche League praxis. A more nuanced analysis is required for this task.

THE EVER-EVOLVING ROLE
OF WESTERN WOMEN

In *The Courage to Be*, Paul Tillich states, "The courage to be oneself is the courage to make of oneself what one wants to be."[2] Yet, if a society pits its ideology against such striving for some while wholeheartedly encouraging it for others, the ability to judge the ethical validity of our acts becomes confused and sometimes paralyzed. As Carl Degler asks, "Must the historic drive for women's individuality stop short of full realization in the name of children, husband, and family?"[3]

Using extensive data, Frances Goldscheider and Linda Waite, authors of *New Families, No Families*, answer Degler with a resounding "No."[4] Goldscheider and Waite discovered that a "revolution is taking place inside the family where changes in sex roles, which have increased women's participation in the paid labor force, are now challenging the rules underlying traditional marriage." This revolution pressures families to change by limiting the time and energy women have available for traditional family tasks.[5]

Historical and social scientific literature is rich in recent studies of this dilemma. My exploration is limited to those factors that most directly relate to this chapter's central question: In what way does woman's biology — that is, the reality that only women can bear children and lactate — relate to the evolution of women's roles in the twentieth century?

From the perspective of anthropology, the family emphasizes community. Throughout most of human experience, the family has functioned as a unit with little or no emphasis on individual goals. The contemporary revolutions in family life, however, are "not the first revolutions in family life. Another dramatic transformation of family life occurred in the nineteenth century when urbanization and industrialization took the production of many goods and services out of the home, leading to the physical separation of men's and women's productive work and to the notion of their lives as separate spheres."[6]

In *Of Woman Born*, feminist Adrienne Rich claims that "the nineteenth- and twentieth-century ideal of the mother and children immured together in the home, the specialization of motherhood for women, the separation of the home from the 'man's world' of wage-earning struggle, ambition, aggression, power, of the 'domestic' from the 'public' or the 'political'" — all are late developments in human history.[7]

The reasons mothers remained at home were complicated and cannot all be explored here, although some major points are worth noting. In most places of work infants and young children could no longer be present because the workplace was not only uncomfortable but noisy and dangerous as well. Furthermore, in the workplace women were looked down on, and, predictably, men received the better-paying and the administrative jobs. In contrast, keeping house, the primary catalyst of domestic comfort, gave women status in the community they could not attain in the workplace. At home, in the days when artificial feeding was dangerous to health and disease prevention primitive, prolonged nursing was a major contributor to a baby's survival. In time the practical necessity of a mother's presence as infant nurturer created an image that was used to define her role.

Although such major technological, economic, and social changes greatly influenced the development of a specialized role for women, new ideologies also shaped their destinies. In *The War over the Family*, Brigitte and Peter Berger analyze these influences. Beginning with the Protestant Reformation, Western culture experienced a major philosophical shift away from a collective focus.

Children could no longer be viewed simply as a part of a family that was in turn part of the larger society. In the past, families functioned to shape children's characters by reproducing cultural patterns, imparting ethical norms, and instilling modes of thought, but as the eighteenth blended into the nineteenth century, the newly emerging American family (especially in the middle classes) centered its attention, energy, and resources on educating children for their own sakes. At first, education focused only on boys. By the middle of the nineteenth century, however, educational and religious leaders urged solicitous attention to the raising of daughters since they would be the mothers and educators of future citizens.

Philosophers, political thinkers, and ministers of religion seized on this image of mothers as the primary educators of the next generation for it solved a major ethical conflict for them. Christian theology for centuries had cautioned against accumulating earthly, material possessions and urged storing up treasure in heaven. At the same time, as a period of rapid economic growth, the nineteenth century produced a new social stratification by wealth and an abundance of material possessions for some individuals. New theological and political principles were needed to explain and justify the erosion of traditional mores in the public sphere. This was accomplished by transferring the maintenance of these values to the domestic sphere and extended to viewing women exclusively in their domestic roles. Having a working wife reduced a man's status in his community. It implied a failure on his part as a provider for his family. Thus, women's role as nurturers of young children expanded into their being guardians of hearth and morality for all society. If this vision of family life was at first confined to the homes of middle-class merchants and artisans, as the nineteenth century progressed, this ideology was diffused to the working classes.[8]

By 1850, however, over a quarter of a million women were working in manufacturing plants in the United States. Also, by the opening of the twentieth century some women had moved, at least as tokens, into all professions. Yet, whether women labored in the factories or argued before the bar, the overwhelming majority of white working women were single. They abandoned work outside the home when they married. By 1920 only 12 percent of professional women were married. This same figure held true through 1940. The reason is easy to comprehend. For married women, work outside the home necessitated two difficult tasks, both arduous and demanding. In every case women were still regarded as the primary child-care parent. For women of the working classes, jobs were most often monotonous, low paying, and without much future. For professional women, their careers most often demanded leaving children to the uncertain care of servants or relatives. The dilemma of all women remains unresolved as long as women, employed or not, are considered the guardians of the hearth, totally responsible for all that occurs in their "domain."

Today, despite the fact that the number of mothers in the workforce is constantly increasing, little has changed in the accepted image of spheres of influence for women and men. Women, even many women with considerable influence in professional circles, continue to bear the responsibility for maintaining the home and raising the children.

In addition, they shoulder the responsibility for maintaining a sense of human connection for all family members. In politics and business, co-operation is always vigorously negotiated, leaving its participants psychologically exhausted and emotionally drained. Since work is often devoid of any true collectivist spirit, employed men and women hope to find all sense of human connection in the home. Many men expect to find such peace without contributing to it, and women perceive themselves as having the obligation to provide it. If this sense of obligation causes a woman to absent herself from the workplace, she often becomes aware of living in a social vacuum cut off from the mainstream of her culture.

Many women experience, as an intense anxiety, a feeling that they are living a life in which their individuality is invisible, even sacrificed, but, at the same time, sense the weight of their responsibilities to others. Tillich recognized the ambiguity inherent in the struggle for individualization and has called for courage in the face of this ambiguity. He writes, "Both self-preservation and self-affirmation logically imply the overcoming of something which, at least potentially, threatens or denies the self. . . . Courage is the power of life to affirm itself in spite of this ambiguity, while the negation of life because of its negativity is an expression of cowardice."[9]

A woman must act. Her family and her self await her decisions. She must decide even knowing that her decisions will be ambiguous, the results uncertain. Some have asked, "Why not return to the traditional family?" They see it as providing for the needs of children and reinforcing adult commitment to family life. Goldscheider and Waite reply that the problems traditional families create are disproportionately accrued by women.[10] Increased life expectancy and decreased fertility mean that homemaking no longer functions as a lifetime career for most women, so many women will choose to combine a professional life with homemaking. Two approaches women take to this combination are "sequencing" professional and home life or working continuously. The mothers who take the latter approach are often perceived as either "real" workers or "mommy trackers," depending on the amount of time and energy they expend in the workplace.

Choosing among these options is an uncertain process. In the past, the new mother may have turned to female relatives for advice. In our century, these family connections are often broken by geography or ideology; however, several new sources of advice and help have appeared in the mid-twentieth century. One is the women's liberation movement. La Leche League is another.

FEMINISM AND MOTHERHOOD

Feminism's understanding of motherhood has been a movement from alienation to rapprochement. Early second-wave feminism abounded in a rejection of motherhood, seeing it as a captivity for women. These early rejectionist themes were followed by a period in which motherhood became an acceptable choice for women. In this second period, emphasis was placed on the necessity and value of shared parenting, including the hope of an equal parenting partnership with a second parent. Today, feminists are exploring motherhood with a new realism. They are discovering that, despite their long struggle to develop an alternative approach to parenting, they are still the primary caregivers, if not in the amount of time spent then in the emotional energy invested.

Since the mid-twentieth century, feminists have searched for an authentic voice about motherhood. Rebecca Chopp states, "Feminist theology is more appropriately termed 'feminist theologies,' for the concerns, issues, and topics addressed vary widely as does the focus of attention and perspective."[11] Chopp perceives four different feminist methods: liberal equalitarianism, romantic expressivism, sectarian separateness, and radical transformism. Feminists employ various approaches to different issues or seek to combine several features from different approaches toward a single issue. Also, at different periods in the evolution of feminism's understanding of motherhood, varying combinations of strategies have been applied among the approaches.

According to feminist writer Ann Snitow, the rejection of motherhood dominated second-wave feminism from approximately 1963 to about 1975.[12] Writings from this time were often liberal egalitarian in tone and put great confidence in Western Enlightenment claims of equality, freedom, and liberty. Many focused on pregnancy and motherhood as a prison. Snitow calls this period the time of the "demon texts" because the writings of this period caused enormous controversy and provided fuel for attacks on feminism in general. In *Inventing Motherhood*, British psychiatrist Ann Dally notes that many of the texts on motherhood from this period emphasized free collective child care and abortion on demand. These writings seldom concerned themselves with any aspect of children's needs. Instead, they focused on the necessity of raising children who were free of sexual stereotypes. It is no wonder that readers of this literature inferred that feminists were antimotherhood.[13]

Some texts spewed out their conviction in hostile language. One such text is Shulamith Firestone's *Dialectic of Sex*. Firestone defines pregnancy as "the temporary deformation of the body of the individual for the sake of the species" and describes childbirth as barbaric, likening it to "shitting a pumpkin."[14] In *Who Cares?: A New Deal for Mothers and Their Small Children*, Penelope Leach notes that a popular magazine had described the full-time care of a baby or small child as "like spending all day, every day, in the exclusive company of an incontinent mental defective."[15] Dally holds that these forceful impressions were probably not true for the majority of feminists and that they obscured much that was valuable and timely in modern feminism.[16]

Snitow believes that many writings in this period were hampered by the inadequate experience and prejudices of their authors and were open to being "demonized, apologized for, endlessly quoted out of context." She observes that these texts engendered both an antifeminist backlash and an intense effort by feminists in all fields to integrate feminism and motherhood. By restricting their focus, Snitow believes, women missed how amazing the early works were in their groundbreaking ideas, particularly that a woman alone could lead a happy, productive, meaningful life.

Early feminist theology also veered away from discussions about mothering. It treated the language of mothering "like a foreign language." Even in Valerie Saiving's classic exploration of love and sin, "The Human Situation: A Feminine View," her personal experiences of motherhood are carefully removed to third-person language. At the time, her existential insights were received as penetrating, but her actual reflections on motherhood went largely unnoticed.[17] In this early period, feminist theologians focused first on the question "Does religion enforce and perpetuate sex-role stereotypes and the power of men over women?" Second, these scholars moved beyond critique to construction of alternatives to sexist theologies. Feminist theologians took a radical transformist position. They rejected the patriarchal names for their experiences and called for a new naming of self and world. They began to realize that only a radical transformation of all human structures — personal, linguistic, cultural, and political — would allow for full human flourishing.

At this point, a tension arose in feminist theology. It reflected distinct perceptions of what was most valuable in women's experience, of the nature of the alienation produced by sexism, of the sources of liberating vision, and of the future toward which feminism was striving. A liberal feminist model held that liberation from oppression was the more potentially transformative experience in women's lives. A traditional model sought to reevaluate women's roles within marriage and motherhood as the key to reforming patriarchal culture. Akin to the traditional model, the romantic expressivist one concentrated on the uniqueness of women's voices. It emphasized what women could bring to society if given full participation in society. This perspective assumed that women's experiences and their voices differed strongly from men's. This approach believed that a harmonious balance in society would occur if men and women could each fully represent their own particularities.[18]

Another dilemma recognized by early feminist theologians was the traditional association of women and nature. There was a growing recognition that humans were becoming alienated from natural processes. The closeness to these processes that women experience through their bodily cycles of menstruation, pregnancy, birth, lactation, and menopause was considered by some feminist authors as a source for revealing to society as a whole its rootedness in nature.[19] Other feminist theologians, such as Judith Plaskow, saw this approach as dangerously close to the traditional equation of women with denigrated nature and men with freedom and spiritual transcendence. Feminist theology would continue to grapple with the difficulty of integrating the new feminist vision with *women's* traditional experiences.

Amid these agonizing dilemmas, the feminist work of exploring motherhood exploded. Feminists began to write books that examined the daily experience of being a mother as well as motherhood's most far-reaching implications. New feminists succeeded in breaking "the [early feminist] taboo on mothers' own descriptions of the fascination and joy of mothering (even in patriarchy) and also the pain, isolation, boredom, murderousness."[20] This period opened up two rival political approaches to motherhood.

Adrienne Rich's *Of Woman Born*, published in 1976, represented one approach. It introduced the task of wresting *mothering* away from *motherhood* as an institution of the patriarchal culture. As Rich perceived it, patriarchal man impregnated "his" wife and expected her to deliver "his" child. Woman's elemental power was reduced to a service she rendered to her child's father. The mother-child relationship, the essential human relationship, was violently altered by the creation of the patriarchal family.[21] Rich's ideology was sectarian separativist in tone. This means she assumed that patriarchal structures are incapable of change and concentrated on the task of creating separate spaces for women. Rich urged women to move toward developing a female culture within which women would support each other and their children without dependence on the uncertain help of the fathers of those children.

Other feminist authors offered an alternative strategy. Their approach was more romantic expressivist in tone. These women argued that as a society we need to open up the joys and responsibilities of "mothering" to men who might then share them with women. These authors also opened up the possibility of fathers as primary caregivers. In such situations, mothers are employed as full-time wage earners while fathers remain at home and take on a full day of child care. Such arrangements were questioned by traditional psychologists. They doubted that fathers could provide the same emotional care to babies and young children as mothers could.[22]

The early 1980s were a transitional period between the hope of equal parenting partnerships and a new realism about how difficult achieving this goal would be. During the 1980s, feminists who supported equal

parenting were able to point to a number of studies that reported benefits resulting from full-time father care.[23] These studies suggested that
fathers who assume full-time child-care responsibilities also shoulder
more household duties than do their counterparts who share no responsibility for child care, these fathers also manage child care in much the
same way as mothers do without losing their sense of masculine identity,
and the emotional and social development of the children in the full-time
care of their fathers does not differ from that of children in the full-time
care of their mothers. These results at least testified to the fact that fathers
as primary caretakers were not emotional disasters. As the 1980s moved
forward into the 1990s, however, women were to discover that not only
was equal parenting hard to achieve, it was also hard to desire. This
passage from feminine control over parenthood to equalitarian fathering and mothering meant women were giving up the special privileges
wound up in the culturally laden word "mother," privileges they would
not instantly regain in the form of freedom and power.

Many contemporary American mothers might tend to describe the
conditions within which they mother as difficult rather than oppressive.
Kathleen Gerson's *Hard Choices* demonstrates that, despite women's
deep commitment to motherhood, their lives are centered less and less
around motherhood and more on a variety of other life issues.

For individual women, most of these issues center on the juggling act
of holding two "jobs" at once. The findings of Arlie Hochschild's *The
Second Shift* contradict the optimism of earlier studies on "co-parenting"
and equalitarian households.[24] According to Hochschild, women continue to carry the majority of domestic responsibilities. Women have also
accepted the total responsibility for maintaining the smooth flow of
daily life. Goldscheider and Waite discovered that even originally equalitarian households experience a pressure to follow more conventional
patterns after the arrival of children.[25]

In the public sphere, it is mostly feminist writers who have taken
responsibility for declaiming the injustice of child-custody laws, the feminization of poverty, the difficulties for women that followed the inception of no-fault divorce, and the inequity of employment. Women are
discouraged by the immensity of their struggles. They have embraced
nurturance as an ethic, and although they sometimes wish but do not
expect that men would share this ethic, women have soldiered on, caring
for their children and continuing to do most of the housework. Many

women feel guilt about neither achieving their feminist goals nor fulfilling their nurturing dreams. Their guilt complicates feminist rage — and slows down feminist activism.[26]

One of the clearest distinctions between contemporary feminist writings and those of the past is confusion in the face of most mothers' failure to fully engage fathers in equal parenting, a goal that seemed achievable in the early 1980s. Traditional role models and workplace pressures often conspire to keep fathers from sharing equally in home responsibilities. Cultural and monetary pressures may also cause fathers to spend time away from the family unit while their children are infants.[27]

Discussions about the "mommy track" reveal another face of this same dilemma. This work trajectory is one that includes time for giving children more attention than current career options allow. This "solution" is the subject of Arlene Cardozo's *Sequencing*. Cardozo explores ways of combining meaningful careers with traditional mothering. Mothers who choose this track first concentrate on establishing themselves in their career fields, then leave full-time employment to focus their energies on full-time child care, and finally become reemployed "through carefully reintegrating their work into their lives so that it enhances rather than dominates their lifestyles."[28] Snitow judges that such ideas as Cardozo's would be revolutionary if society rethought work for everyone. Instead, "this corporate plan became a symbol of the continuing divide between male and female life-stories — with motherhood the signpost at the crossroads."[29] In an effort to close this gap, many feminists are now constructing their demands for parental leaves and custody decisions in "gender-neutral" language.[30]

Feminist theologian Bonnie Miller-McLemore's *Also a Mother* is a full exploration of women's roles in both work and family as a theological issue. It is also a premier example of the new realism in feminist thought. Miller-McLemore recognizes that beneath the middle-class scuffle over gender roles and child care lies an essential religious crisis of work and life, of generativity and care. Although it might be simpler to ponder "work" or "love" or even "the family" in isolation, as sometimes has been the case in theology, these three arenas are integrally related.

Miller-McLemore encourages feminist theologians to add the relevant ethical and theological analysis to feminism's continuing analysis of the social, political, and economic context surrounding the evolving life of the family. She also seeks to remain aware of the many "women whose gifts are buried or aborted" by the overwhelming burden of the double shift, a burden increased by the fantasy of the perfect mother, who assumes the responsibility of total provision for emotional, social, and intellectual development of all family members.

Women are swept up with men in the detrimental changes occurring in paid employment. Expectations that technology would lighten human workloads have proven overly optimistic. Instead, there is an increasing pressure to produce more. As Miller-McLemore observes, "The infamous Protestant work ethic of the Puritans has degenerated from a view of work as a means to ensure the well-being of the human community to an excuse to seek one's own personal profit." The end result is a piety and a cultural context that condone "self-righteous individual achievement, selfish self-sufficiency, and ruthless ambition."[31]

The postindustrial economy would have put the nuclear family under increasing stress with or without a feminist critique. Goldscheider and Waite argue that American society confronts the choice between creating "new families" or being left with no families at all. Their studies of young, not-yet-married adults suggest that leaving family roles much as they have been since the 1950s will result in "fewer and fewer adults who are willing to fill them."[32] Neither young men nor young women are discovering cultural models that would demonstrate a way to integrate children into a life that is both fulfilling and equalitarian.

Miller-McLemore advances Barbara Katz Rothman's cultural analysis that regards the deeply ingrained ideologies of patriarchy, technology, and capitalism as determining how we think about work and about intimate relationships. These ideologies interweave to form the infrastructures of a high-tech, product-oriented "commodification of life." This infrastructure punishes "women who choose procreation and nurturance over production alone" and at the same time discourages "men from becoming more than marginally involved in activities that give and sustain life."[33]

For Miller-McLemore, feminist theology needs to engage productively in a wide-ranging discussion of family life on the basis of a reappraisal of the theological definitions of love and work. Many women have been overlooked by the churches where "the term *family values* has become a distorted and sometimes politically dangerous code word for reinstituting male dominance and female self-sacrifice."[34] Feminist theologians, also, have overlooked many women. They have focused their attack on the use of biblical narratives that portray women as the source of evil, at the effects of always naming God as male, and at the way women are excluded from church leadership. Although these are worthwhile goals, they affect only indirectly the challenges in the domestic sphere. Women are caught between two ideals of womanhood, neither of which adequately explains what it means to be female. In an interview about her original groundbreaking essay, Valerie Saiving stated that she never claimed a universal ground of womanhood. Instead, she held that the essay stressed the importance of "where you are when you do your theology." What it means to be female will "not be found either in biology or in socialization but in some dialectical relationship between the two." Biology limits, but it does not dictate, who we can be. Because women and only women bear children and are capable of lactation, motherhood in reality or in possibility is one of the "limits" with which women must contend.[35] Reflection on motherhood, however, must also take into consideration three other important factors. Simply becoming a mother biologically does not render a woman a nurturing person. The complex experience that is "mothering" can be performed by persons not the child's actual mother. Adoption is an example. And while bearing children and nursing them may significantly affect a woman's development, even if she has a large family, pregnancy and lactation are but part of her life. Who a woman is and what she contributes to the common good may owe a great deal to what she learned from mothering. Thus, even women who are never employed outside the home are called to be full members of the community at large.

Redefining women's and men's roles in the workplace community demands a redefinition of their roles within the family. This project is far from complete, but it cannot be abandoned, for the family is a precious resource, one that can be lost simply because as a society we focus too little of the right kinds of attention on it. Because more feminists have begun to recognize the complexity of the issues confronting the family, the period of new realism is only just beginning.

REDEFINING THE NEEDS OF CHILDREN

An integral part of the feminist discussion of motherhood is a scrutiny of the traditional wisdom regarding the needs of children. The way a society meets the needs of its children is a deeply theological issue. Decisions in this area reflect the moral perceptions of individuals and of the culture as a whole. Challenging traditional understandings of children's needs demands a new look at the traditional meaning of distributive justice, charity as ordered love, and *agape* as self-sacrificing love.

Very early second-wave feminism realized that what the culture understood to be the authentic needs of children conflicted with what women were beginning to perceive as their own needs. Men assumed that their own needs, such as opportunities for paid employment, would not conflict with the culturally defined needs of children. Women, however, did see a conflict and called for an examination of the authentic needs of children in light of this dilemma.

The temptation of society as a whole is to assume that children must need only what it seems possible to give them. For some early feminists, this meant that traditionally defined needs that conflicted with needs of women must not be authentic needs of children, but, as the new realism takes hold, the feminist examination of children's needs reflects its new realism about family life as a whole. In this regard, feminists concede that children's authentic needs might conflict with women's valid objectives.

Writing in 1981, Ann Dally focused her critique on the strictures of child-care professionals. Dally censured mid-twentieth-century literature on child care as unrealistic and overdemanding of mothers. Women, she believed, were defrauded by a patriarchal culture intent on confining them in the home. She did not argue with the claim that children need hands-on nurturing but with the assertion that the best person to care for a baby or small child is the mother because mothers have a mothering instinct. Such a claim entitled the child to the exclusive care of his or her mother and held that even a short separation might be damaging. The physicians, psychologists, and other advisors who advocated this system blamed all physical and psychological problems a child might have on his or her mother's care.

Dally acknowledged that a child's environment is a key factor in development and that a child's parents are major contributors to that environment. Her writing reflects a hope that the answer to the child-care dilemma will be found in shared parenting. She further held that the best mothers understand what they can and cannot be to their child and how they mesh as a person with the needs of the baby. Such mothers know when to delegate or relinquish certain child-care functions. Thus, those goods that a child truly needs from his mother do not require her constant presence. A child's real needs are unconditional love, continuity and reliability, protection from areas of the community with which he or she cannot yet cope, and a clear understanding of what activities and opportunities are appropriate to each age.

Dally also questioned the existence of maternal instinct. She observed that, whereas many women do form strong feelings of involvement with their infants, many other women do not. The reasons mothers become attached to their children are multiple and complex. Postulating some universal maternal instinct, Dally argued, confuses the issue.[36]

Dally believes that fathers can parent as well as mothers and that there is no necessary difference in their approach to parenting. Their roles can be interchangeable. Many feminist psychologists agree with Dally's perceptions. They hold that limiting a baby's intimate exposure to one other person divides the development of attachment and separation along gender lines, rendering girls more accomplished at the former and boys better at the latter.[37]

Recently, feminist realism has begun to question the stance that Dally expressed. In *The Mother Zone*, Marni Jackson explores this same territory from the point of view of personal experiences. She places the question of instinct within the context of the intimate triad of father, mother, and child formed when a baby is born.[38] She finds that neither a totally analytical feminist viewpoint nor a sentimental traditional one captures the sum and substance of the early parenting experiences. What she sees is a bit of biology interacting with a lot of choice. Jackson writes that mothers are nine months ahead of fathers in forging a bond with their babies. Even after the father finally is able to actually hold his child, the mother and father have different roles to play at first. Jackson sees the mother's task almost from the beginning as that of separating herself from her baby. Sooner or later, even if she is breast-feeding, a mother must "extricate herself from the baby bubble." Because the father can determine how much or how little he will do with the infant, his task differs from that of the mother. He and the baby both lose if he slips into letting the mother decide how he constructs his own zone of care. Yet, because mothers are socialized in nurturance since childhood, they may find it easy to do everything. Jackson relates that after their son was born, her husband continued to take his accustomed lengthy showers, whereas she "could shower so quickly that the mirror didn't fog and the backs of my knees stayed dry."[39]

For Miller-McLemore these varying observations by feminist mothers demonstrate that it is time to shift to the next wave of feminism. How does she envision this new wave? First, we must face up fully to the reality that, until recently, mothers and their children have been pushed to the fringes by the society as a whole. Second, we have to realize that issues concerning mothers and children have come to the forefront but that this does not spell the demise of feminism. For, as Elizabeth Schussler Fiorenza states, "Children are not just the responsibility of mothers, not even just the responsibility of both parents. Their rights are given into the care of all of us, not because we are women but because they are our future."[40]

Like most mothers, states Susan Moller Okin in *Justice, Gender, and the Family*, feminists recognize that given beneficial circumstances, child care can be both delightful and challenging. For this reason, she asserts, shared parenting ought to remain a major feminist goal. It is necessary for justice between the sexes. Child care is so time consuming that if one person is left to do it single-handedly, he or she is prevented from pursuing many other social goods. Okin insists that small-scale loving day care can be a positive experience for children. In addition, if day care is subsidized by government funding, it "can help to alleviate the obstacle that the inequality of family circumstance poses for equality of opportunity."[41]

But is day care really good for children? Sandra Scarr notes, "The idea that babies and young children can be successfully reared apart from their parents both horrifies and fascinates American parents."[42] Caught between the child specialists who insist on maternal care and their very real professional and economic needs, these parents feel trapped in a catch-22 situation. She holds that parents ought to think in terms of age-appropriate care. For infants this means frequent interaction with loving familiar adults. Studies on institutionalized children have demonstrated that even when these children were given adequate physical care, they were emotionally and psychologically unhealthy and often unable to cope with adult life. While such studies concluded that these children suffered from "maternal deprivation," Scarr believes such conclusions were structured by societal expectations that mothers were the natural caretakers of their children. She concludes that these children actually suffered the broader deprivation of appropriate human contact, not "maternal" deprivation. She reasons that care by someone other than the mother needs to be judged by its quality, not simply by the fact that someone other than the mother has tended the child. She contends that good child care fits into the work and care patterns of the child's family and of the family's larger society.

When Miller-McLemore looks at the child-care situation, her conclusions are more radically transformist than Scarr's earlier ones. Miller-McLemore holds that children's needs cannot be met without vast changes in societal priorities. She points out that in today's market economy, when men and women work out visions of adulthood, children are too often viewed first as desirable possessions and then as burdens because they limit us. She offers a biblical and theological reflection that challenges this view. She turns to Genesis 33:13–14, the passage in which Jacob adjusts the pace of his journey so that a hardship will not be worked on the more slowly moving children. She also evokes the image of Jesus rebuking adults for keeping children at a distance from him. By his rebuke Jesus communicates that something about children identifies what it means to be an "ideal member" of the new religious movement that is defined by lack of worldly power.[43]

Miller-McLemore postulates that factoring in "the pace of children" when we plan our adult lives would reshape contemporary views of work and care. Giving more time to be present with children would return gifts to us. With them we could give ourselves fully to the joy and activity of the moment without past regrets or anxieties about tomorrow. Combining the pressures and commitments of adult life with living according to the pace of children can also cause tedium and stress. Despite these difficulties, children bring a vitality into adult lives. We gain a renewed investment in our world and our community. We bring some of the joy and awe our children inspire to our own endeavor to contribute to the world. Children can also revitalize the spiritual life of any adult. "Genuine care of a small being demands finely tuned 'metaphysical attitudes,' which I would identify as the same significant moral and religious virtues long upheld by biblical and religious traditions; the priority of holding over acquiring; humility and profound sense of one's limits; humor and resilient cheerfulness amid the realities of life; respect for persons; responsiveness to growth; and ultimately, the capacity for what Ruddick calls 'attentive love.'"[44] To Okin's argument that justice between genders requires shared parenting, Miller-McLemore adds that, when society effectively bars men from meaningful parenting tasks, they are deprived of a vital moral and spiritual experience.

The question remains, "Just what do children need? What is attentive care?" Miller-McLemore stresses that children do not need the kind of self-sacrificing love that is often esteemed as the Christian ideal. In fact, love for the children in our care can never be disinterested. It is impossible to separate what we give from what we receive. The good parent is no more saint or hero than is the good spouse. Even in early infancy, when a baby needs almost constant nurturing, she gives her parents the gift of caring for her. Therefore, we ought not confuse genuine parenting with unconditional maternal self-sacrifice. When we do so, we deprive the child of the attentive love of others who genuinely care for him. This other care also allows the baby's mother time for renewal that absorption in her own work provides. Such renewal enriches her love for her child.

In this call for a more balanced approach to meeting a child's needs, Miller-McLemore places her theological reflection within the feminist model, but she differs from many earlier feminists when she insists that children are immensely more valuable, more vulnerable, and a lot more work "than our cultural imagination has conceded." Some aspects of parenting are both everyday and lifelong commitments. Children need to belong to a particular family, in which the attachments of the first few years are pivotal to a child's growth; however, neither the everyday nor the lifelong commitment is given to the mother, or even to both parents, alone. Our children have been given by God not only to their parents but to the community as a whole. Children do not grow linearly from early complete attachment to mother to later independence in the midst of the broader community. As they grow they evolve new and more adequate ways of relating to relatives, neighbors, peers, parents of peers, and a variety of unrelated adults.

Miller-McLemore believes that American reluctance to expand day care rests on the belief that it is mothers who are ultimately responsible for their own children. Americans fail to ask about their responsibility to any but their own children (if they have any). When most people have no firsthand experience with what it means to be involved in the immediate context of child care, they become unable to "extend the instinct of life preservation beyond themselves to the next generation." Reserving child care for mothers alone robs nonmothers of "a great training ground" for learning an ethic that does not pit justice against care but encompasses both. To exclude fathers and nonparents from early child care "is to lose a precious resource and negate a viable avenue of full humanhood."[45]

In the spirit of the new feminist realism, Miller-McLemore and others call for a radical reevaluation of the needs of infants and young children that extends far beyond earlier hopes for shared parenting. Infants, they claim, do not need the exclusive care of their mothers. From their earliest days, a variety of interrelationships provides infants with optimum growth opportunities.[46] Furthermore, they insist, restricting infant and early childhood care to mothers robs other adults of a vital life experience. It also restricts the mother's opportunities for self-fulfillment. This, in turn, deprives her infant of the care of a more fulfilled, less emotionally drained mother.

It is perhaps La Leche League's most deeply held tenet that the physical, emotional, and psychological health of the baby and the mother depend on an early period of mother-infant proximity that sets the organization most at loggerheads with the hopes of second-wave feminism. Yet, while we can never ignore this important conflict, it is also important to acknowledge how often feminists and League advocates walk the same sacred paths of women's ways of knowing and acting.

chapter 5

. . . .

Challenging the Public Domain from within the Private Sphere

Every word published in La Leche League material, as well as every word uttered in its meetings and conferences, reveals the depth of its belief in its mission to promote "good mothering through breastfeeding."

A CENTRAL CONCEPT: MOTHER-INFANT PROXIMITY

A foundational ideal of La Leche League's work is a deep, abiding belief that a child's healthy development depends on an early physical closeness with its mother. The League endorses Ashley Montague's concept that an infant's earliest months might actually be called a second period of gestation.[1]

The early members of La Leche League were mobilized into action by their belief that bottle feeding placed an emotional distance between a baby and its mother that would cause a loss of the symbiotic relationship between mother and child. This central concern led the League into many other issues of mothering. From the League's point of view, the need for mother-baby closeness begins in the hospital. The third edition of the League's manual urged mothers to insist regularly that they did not want their babies to be given bottles of water or formula in the nursery and that they needed to nurse their infants very frequently. Rooming in, a practice that allows the mother to have the baby in her room for all or most of the time, was highly recommended by the League.

Keeping the infant close is important because it encourages the frequent feedings that are necessary if breast feeding is to be maintained. Jan Riordan and Kathleen Auerbach explain in *Breastfeeding and Human Lactation* that the fact of breast-feeding babies needing frequent feedings often causes alarm in uninformed mothers. The breast-fed infant feeds both more frequently than and in patterns that differ from those of bottle-fed babies, whose feedings are often regulated by external factors like the clock and the relatively less digestible curds of artificial baby milk. On the other hand, the newborn breast-fed baby may feed frequently in a pattern known as "cluster feedings." These constitute a series of minifeedings, which can be seen as courses in the larger banquet that is the single breast-feeding episode.[2]

While La Leche League proposes that mothers remain within full-time reach of their infants as a practical technique to avoid resorting to bottle feeding and all its inherent difficulties, this is only one of many reasons La Leche League insists on mother-baby proximity. The League sees the baby's first weeks of life as a time when "a baby's wants are a baby's needs" and when "no timetable can tell you how often you should nurse your baby."[3] The baby simply needs to be close to its mother most of the time, whether awake or sleeping. For the League mother, she was her baby's world.

Originally, La Leche League mothers grounded this belief in their own experience and on the beliefs of Drs. Ratner and White as well as on those of behavioral scientist Niles Newton. Later, they found additional support in much of the literature on child care and parenting available in the mid-twentieth century. One book the League recommended for both its philosophy and its readability was Louise Kaplan's *Oneness and Separateness*.

La Leche League praised Kaplan's book and recommended it at meetings because it underlined the importance of mother-infant togetherness and sensitively portrayed why and how a mother's presence and understanding, as well as her unconditional, unscheduled love, were necessary for maximum development of the child.[4] According to Kaplan, a psychologist, "In the first three years of life every human being undergoes yet a second birth, in which he is born as a psychological being possessing selfhood and separate identity. The quality of self an infant achieves in those crucial three years will profoundly affect all of his subsequent existence."[5]

With these words Kaplan stated what has been for many twentieth-century Western parents, within and outside La Leche League, the concept that, more than any other, guides the choices they make as they raise their children. Kaplan's elaboration of this central concept, however, might not find such universal adherence. She insisted that in a *normal* infancy, every child uses his or her *mother* as a beacon of orientation. Kaplan bases her claims on her own interpretation of the research done by Margaret Mahler. In 1959, Mahler began a study of the development of selfhood by observing the interactions of babies and mothers on a continuous daily basis. This research led to the theory that a mother's consistent presence is vital for providing the child with a secure base from which to explore the world, a prerequisite for the healthy development of a separate identity. Mahler also hypothesized that many psychological disorders that typify the pathology of our society originate in weaknesses in the separation-individuation process.[6]

Such findings and theories belong to a consistent body of thought that includes the work of Anna Freud and Erik Erikson. The focus is over and over again on the central importance of a mother's presence to her child. What emerges is a twofold understanding. The quality of child care in the first three years of life is pivotal for both child and adult development. Also, there is one certain way to assure that the child receives a good beginning — infants and young children need to spend the majority of their time during those years in the guiding presence of a loving and consistent mother. The goal is individuation, which is the separation of the child from the mother as a whole, healthy, and unique personality ready to take his or her first steps toward full independence. Such independence is possible only if the child is not thrust into it too soon or too abruptly. Although periods of maternal absence are a necessary part of the development process, these absences need to be appropriate to the child's developmental readiness. They should be lengthened only gradually and sometimes abandoned when the child experiences a need to retreat a little to an earlier developmental stage. The whole process is orchestrated by the perceived needs of the child.

Kaplan recognized that there were controversies about infant and child development and that readers were likely to ask, "How do we know this?" Therefore, the book contains extensive notes on the various points of controversy and on some of the studies done in the field of child development. League philosophy concurred with Kaplan on the need for early mother-infant symbiosis. In fact, objections to this conviction were met with censure as expressed in reviews of child-care literature that argued against this principle. "The experts give such conflicting, often outrageous opinions, one is again grateful for the basic good common parent-sense we in La Leche League have come to value. Of particular note is the rather blatant disregard for a baby's needs."[7]

Both League literature and Kaplan's work suggest that women are being deprived of the full mothering experience that is rightfully theirs. Kaplan found it ironic that "the vital importance of a human infant's *attachment* to his mother should be subverted by shame and impatience at the very moment in history when the complaints of human *detachment* are the loudest." She firmly believed that rather than concentrate all our attention on social forces as the source of the contemporary disequilibrium, we need to focus again on the importance of the "biological origins of our longings for human attachment." Another important tenet of Kaplan's theory is her perception that human nature is universal. She held that all humans share an attachment to some fixed point, a home base, from which the rest of their lives radiate.[8] In her writing and in League understanding, no consideration is given to the concept that this "home base" might be a matrix of loving, involved persons rather than just the mother. Kaplan's conclusions demonstrate a glaring gap, as her research and writing predate most postmodern gender studies.

In healthy development, Kaplan maintains, the child goes through a series of reconciliations from birth to about his third birthday. She envisions these as cycles of "breaking free and returning to base" in a series of events she calls "our second birth." She divides these "events" into rough time periods: (1) "the beginnings," birth to six weeks; (2) "oneness," four weeks to five months; (3) "beginning separation and early conquests," four months to eleven months; (4) "love affair with the world," ten months to eighteen months; and (5) "the new beginning," fifteen months to three years. There exist affinities between La Leche League philosophy and the full scope of Kaplan's theory of child development from birth to three years. The League's close adherence to these concepts is an important factor in its ethic of infant care.

La Leche League deems the weeks immediately following birth, Kaplan's first stage, or "the beginnings," as particularly important. League leaders advise new mothers to think of the first four to six weeks as an adjustment period, "a time of getting to know each other."[9] For the mother, the new relationship holds out an opportunity for a re-creation of herself, an expansion, a change for the better. Kaplan worries that today's mothers are at risk because so many expectations are placed on them that they may feel incapable of meeting their infant's needs. One of the League's founders remembers sitting by her crying baby's cradle, feeling at a loss for what to do. As a new mother, she felt put out at the turn of events, at herself, and at her baby.[10]

What mothers need to see, Kaplan asserts, is that the baby, too, has his part. The infant arrives with a "biological readiness" to employ his surroundings to his best advantage. The more a mother has come to know her baby, the stronger the mother-baby attachment, the better the baby's chances of emotional survival. For La Leche League mothers the breast-feeding experience is often one that overcomes both any helplessness they may feel faced with an infant's needs and even any previously held resistance to the mothering role.

Lyn Abruzzi was a senior in college, planning to go on for a master's degree, when she unexpectedly became pregnant. Although she was unhappy to be pregnant, she and her husband accepted it, resolving to allow Lyn to pursue a satisfying life for herself by combining school and part-time mothering. She chose to breast-feed her son, convinced that "without the easy necessary closeness between mother and child that nursing brings, my motherly instincts, so deeply buried within me, would have emerged . . . less fully."[11]

Early in infancy, a baby moves steadily away from a preoccupation with the events inside her body to the beginnings of an outer awareness. One of the first signs is that her smile becomes increasingly stimulated by specifically human sights and sounds. By the end of this period, the mother notices that the baby who had seemed to look "right through her" now recognizes her face. In fact, the baby seeks eye-to-eye contact. Kaplan sees this interplay between mother and child as the earliest of human dialogues, in which exist "the potentials for all later erotic, verbal and cultural dialogue between one human adult and another."[12]

A League mother expressed these same feelings in poetry:

Bound, child, inextricably to your mother,
    First umbilically,
Then warmly, to soft breasts.
    By eyes, watching in protection,
    By arms, clasping.
    By love — eternally.

Child, laughing up at my breast,
May your laughter be forever repeated
    In your father's eyes.[13]

In many traditional societies, infants are soothed and comforted; crying is understood as expressing a need that is quickly met. In twentieth-century America, however, this earliest dialogue does not always go so smoothly. The contemporary practice of expecting babies to spend most of their hours in cribs and carriages imposes a disconnection from the mother's body that leaves modern newborns with only crying to signal their need for contact with their mother. Further, many parents leave the baby to cry for fear of "spoiling" her. Ironically, the baby who cries a lot may not be considered a "good" baby, but he will receive more attention than a more self-sufficient infant.

These conditions render the infant's entrance into human dialogue more stormy than it is for babies in traditional societies. La Leche League often advises its mothers to look to traditional societies for models of good mothering. One League mother living in Africa relates hearing occasional comments indicating that many Africans thought Europeans could not nurse their infants. In her own experience, she found that mothering her second child in Nigeria and her third child in Ghana were much more positive experiences than that of mothering her first child in Bloomington, Illinois. In Africa, all infant crying tends to be interpreted as a signal that the baby is hungry. Thus, it was easy for her to follow a demand schedule. In fact, in Nigeria, when her daughter Ingred was small, people sitting near her in a church service or meeting often said, "Nurse her, nurse her."[14]

Another factor is at work in this early mother-baby dialogue. Breast-feeding mothers are aided by the hormone oxytocin, which promotes lactation and stimulates a receptive attitude that helps mothers identify and empathize with their infants. Nursing is not necessary to establish the dialogue, but it helps mothers overcome resentment that interrupted sleep patterns and the frequent demands of the newborn generate. For Kaplan, nursing serves as a tool for establishing "emotional availability." Getting to know his or her mother prepares the infant for psychological oneness with her, a oneness that is necessary before the infant can begin to discover separateness.[15]

Kaplan's next stage, four weeks to five months, or "oneness," is a movement toward an intensity of closeness between mother and baby. At the close of this stage,

> The baby now has a specific attachment to a specific mother. He will play out the drama of becoming a separate and unique self with this *one* human partner and with no other person. His father plays a significant role in the drama, but until separateness is achieved the father's part is confined to a subplot that enriches and fills out the basic mother-infant relationship. . . .
>
> The special relationship the infant shares with his mother must be flexible enough to include love for others. It must be strong enough to bear the strain of the child's struggles to become a self. Above all, the specific attachment to the mother must hold together when the awful fact of separateness finally dawns on the child. . . . Whenever . . . the world frustrates his effort to conquer it, the child will long to restore the primary bliss of . . . being an angel baby in the lap of a Madonna.[16]

Here is perhaps one of the strongest examples of Kaplan's determination to see human nature as universal and grounded in biology. She has stated that biology has been ignored in our search for the social causes of contemporary human afflictions. Yet, despite her comparison of traditional and modern societies, she comes close to ignoring the social in favor of the biological. In doing so, she fails to see mothers in the full context of their environments, whether traditional or Western middle-class. The human activities of nursing and birthing are never far removed from the ways in which they are interpreted in specific social and political contexts. In both cultures, even in the 1970s, it was mothers who performed most of the child care. No comparative studies are offered of situations in which fathers or other caregivers share child-care responsibilities with the mother on an equal basis or act as primary caregiver. Nor does Kaplan consider situations in which there are no fathers as household providers to allow mothers to be with their infants full-time. And despite calls to look to traditional societies for models of child care, both Kaplan and the League neglect to note that babies in most of these societies are raised in an extended family household where infants need not cry because so many persons exist to meet their needs.

Yet her conclusions sound universal, which is how La Leche League understood them. For the League, to bypass this mode of mothering was to leave one's child psychologically and emotionally vulnerable. Founding mother Mary Ann Cahill urges a mother to develop a "maternal sensor" so that she can pick up her baby's message: " 'Mom, I need you. You're my water wings in this deep ocean of a world. When you leave, I'm over my head and I'm floundering.' "[17] To the founding mothers, leaving an infant or toddler on a regular basis or for a lengthy period of time was neglect of a mother's obligation to love her child. They uncritically took for granted that a mother could find gratification in spending her days with children, living at a pace completely harmonized to that of infants and toddlers. Such assurance was grounded in their own experiences.

To understand La Leche League, one must be fully aware of the centrality of mother-baby proximity as a driving force behind much of the League's work. It is equally important, however, to realize that this principle is not held as an inflexible commandment. Rather, it is an ideal that no mother achieves perfectly. La Leche League has always conceded that full-time mothering is not possible for all mothers. At the same time, the League strongly urges mothers to be sure their reasons for leaving an infant are vital ones. League leaders frequently have been directed to be cautious in their responses to mothers who intend to be away from home on a regular basis. Leaders are reminded that, although the League hopes that a working or student mother will come to assent to its theories, she is welcome at meetings even if she does not. Each individual mother's final decision is undoubtedly based on a complex set of reasons, both acknowledged and unacknowledged. She may initially attend meetings only to learn about the mechanics of breast feeding. The leader, however, will have a different agenda. Her goal is to make the employed or student mother feel accepted so she will continue attending League meetings. This is seen as the League's best chance to get across its principle of mother-baby proximity.[18]

MOTHER CARE, OTHER CARE

Within La Leche League beliefs, there is a sharp division between two types of other-care givers. The father is in a class by himself, and then there is everyone else. The role of the father within the League family is explored at length later in this chapter. At this point my focus is on those potential caregivers whom the League understands as being outside the family circle. They include relatives, friends, and those employed to help in child care.

When considering the question, "With whom could I leave my baby?" League literature is most apt to insist, "With no one." Relatives are perceived to have a role in the new baby's life, but not as primary or even secondary caregivers. They are encouraged to demonstrate their concern and love for the baby by helping the mother in other ways: "If friends or relatives offer to help, explain that you can manage the baby's care, but an extra pair of hands is always welcome with the older children or the ever-present dishes in the sink and laundry in the hamper."[19] In the League's early years, La Leche League mothers ran into a generation gap when older relatives cared for their babies. The new mother might find that her own mother would insist on giving the baby bottles because she did not trust that breast milk could be fully nourishing.

As to employing someone to care for the baby while the mother engaged in other activities, the League urged mothers to look at their plans from a long-range perspective. There are two circumstances that might result in the mother's wishing to leave the baby. One is the house-bound, childbound feeling that overwhelms all mothers. The League offers two ways to approach this situation. The mother should first look at it from the baby's point of view. The manual pointed out that a baby has no sense of time. To be left at all, from a baby's perspective, is to be abandoned. The manual acknowledged that mothers do, of course, have needs but urged them to realize that, because of their maturity, they are better equipped to postpone them. League literature fails to consider that the baby left in the care of a nurturing familiar person may not feel abandoned at all. League mothers remain dubious of child-development specialists who hold that the lessons of history and common sense suggest that children have thrived in the care of persons other than their mothers throughout history.

Leader Nance Hahn noted, "Many feminists believe that our culture assumes that maternal love should be totally selfless. Yet, when a League mother prioritizes her infant's immediate needs over what she sees as her own more remote needs and desires, she does not consider this self-sacrifice because she believes that her own, as well as the baby's well being, is enhanced by this choice." Hahn saw the years when her children were infants, toddlers, preschoolers, and primary schoolers as a small slice of time in her life as the adult. For her children, on the other hand, they were "everything." She chose full-time, total-immersion mothering as her profession while her children were young, and she loved it. She felt that she might someday opt for a midlife career change and become employed outside the home. But, in the meantime, she was happy with rewards that were more private, more personal, and less tangible.[20]

Second, League mothers believe that breast-fed babies can go everywhere, even places where bottle feeding would be difficult, because, from the nursing mother's point of view, breast feeding entails no equipment and the supply is unending. Mothers tell of nursing in restaurants, in doctors' offices, in church, and at sporting events. One English mother, Lynne Emerson, reported that breast feeding was especially important when her car broke down in a blizzard and a ten-minute car trip turned into an all-day ordeal.[21]

BREAST FEEDING AND
THE EMPLOYED MOTHER

The question of leaving the baby is, however, more challenging when the mother is considering returning to work outside the home. The League takes a variety of stances on the role of outside employment for mothers. An entire chapter of the League manual and many articles in League newsletters are devoted to helping the employed mother breast-feed. The first solution offered is usually to consider taking the baby to work. References to care providers are always cautionary. The League emphasizes, "A baby needs a loving, nurturing person, and this person should be the same someone, not an often changing parade of new faces and personalities."[22] This is not a unique perspective, but the League insists that, even if such a sitter is found, there is a danger that the baby will transfer his or her primary attachment to the caretaker. In addition, the manual warns that even the best of sitters has priorities other than the mother's child. The caretaker may move or take another job. This not only is disrupting for the mother but represents a serious loss of a loved one for the child. Problems surrounding the uncommitted or erratic child-care worker are cultural characteristics of our mobile contemporary Western culture. Such problems certainly do challenge today's family, but the League departs from the feminist new realists in expecting mothers, not society at large, to step into the breach.

Some League mothers believe a woman can be content when her lifelong role is that of wife, mother, and homemaker. Founding mother Mary White declares, "I don't see why a woman needs any other career than that of wife and mother. It's the most fulfilling one there is."[23]

Opinion on this issue is not monolithic. Not all League members believe that mothering is the only career most women would ever need. Of these members many would agree with Hahn that the best solution is for a mother to place her nonmothering career on a back burner while her children are young. Some of the best expressions of this understanding are contained in *What's a Smart Woman Like You Doing at Home?* Although the work does not carry the imprimatur of La Leche League, it, like Kaplan's book, is carried in the League's catalog and is often mentioned at meetings. The authors of this book are women who tried mothering while working outside the home and gave up their careers. The reasons they chose to do so were varied, but they made a common discovery once they had made their decision. They found unexpected richness and self-fulfillment in their new lives as mothers. Editor Linda Burton relates that she spent her twenties searching for fulfillment in what many might consider glamorous jobs — as an actress, as a fundraiser, and as a public relations writer. But it was at home, in the underrated profession of wife and mother, that she finally found fulfillment.[24] Statements like Burton's challenge the claim that women who remain at home will go stale and that homemaking lacks stimulation. Despite the widely held currency of such views, some feminist writers relate experiences demonstrating that each situation is individual and that many women who "passionately love" their children nonetheless found "no room for simply being themselves" when they were full-time mothers.[25]

Personal desires aside, the solution of taking a break from paid employment is not financially possible for all mothers. In the face of this economic reality, League mothers have offered two approaches to such situations. The first is to develop an economic lifestyle that minimizes the need for both parents to work. The second is to offer ways to combine motherhood and employment in a way that encourages giving the young baby's needs the highest priority. Each approach found expression in books published by the League in the mid-1980s.

In *The Heart Has Its Own Reasons*, Mary Ann Cahill brought together narratives of League families who overcame the financial crunch without the mother's returning to outside employment. The book remains basically a practical guide to living on one salary, no matter how small. Some narratives reported major lifestyle changes. The Schilkes of Georgia built a home from salvage. And although Mary Ellen Schilke conceded that it was rough living, she truly believed the sacrifice was well worth the blessing of being able to stay at home while her children were young.[26]

Most accounts in the book dealt with smaller efforts, such as careful menu planning, saving on heating and transportation costs, smart and creative approaches to clothing a family, and family-created entertainment. The mothers who shared their stories with Cahill found that these efforts added up, when measured against the costs of being employed, to savings that allowed them to stay at home. This was not a book about frugality for its own sake. The value was mother-baby proximity. The mothers' efforts were fueled by the realization that, as one mother, Ruth Faux, put it, "Babies don't wait to grow up."

Other League mothers find that remaining unemployed is not a possibility. Kaye Lowman is a mother of four, a longtime League leader, the author of the League's history, *The LLLove Story*, and a successful freelance publisher. In her book *Of Cradles and Careers: A Guide to Reshaping Your Job to Include a Baby in Your Life*, she wrote, "Many women wait in vain for the right moment to set aside their careers in favor of starting a family — a time that for many women simply never comes." Yet throughout her book runs the theme that mother-baby separation is a secondary choice. She discovered that the ways mothers found to minimize separation were many and varied. The reason for doing so, however, was uniformly the same: the realization that babies need to be with their mothers, and mothers need to be with their babies.

The book contains numerous narratives of women who confronted this dilemma in a variety of creative ways. One approach included ways of developing a reduced work schedule such as permanent part-time, job sharing, and longer maternity leaves. The second major solution these mothers employed was to bring baby and workplace together, either by choosing self-employment or by bringing the baby to the place of employment — or by combining the two.

Lowman was especially positive about one aspect of careers for mothers: "An interesting thing happened on the day mother walked out the door to go to work. On the way down the front walk she brushed shoulders with dad, who had come home to claim his rightful place in the mainstream of family life." Despite the metaphorical language used here, her findings reveal what appeared to be a real change in the infrastructure of the American family. "As we analyzed the information from the hundreds of women who shared their experiences with us for this book, one fact became increasingly evident: These dual career couples are truly sharing, working together as a team, to make a home and raise their children."[27]

Such an analysis reveals a striking evolution in La Leche League thought about the working mother. Although Lowman's statement, written in 1984, lacked the new realism about the dual-career family discussed in the previous chapter, it did reveal the lack of rigidity in League principles regarding women's roles. This link to feminism did not suddenly appear in the last decade. It was always there in the League's belief that women could change the culture. This principle was apparent in its challenge to the medical profession, in its worldwide struggle for improved infant nutrition, in its nontraditional understanding of father-mother role divisions, and in the strength of its woman-to-woman network.

LINKS TO FEMINISM

Dr. Herbert Ratner, the editor of *Child and Family*, who called himself La Leche League's "Socratic midwife," saw the League as distinguished from the feminist movement. He held that the League was grounded in the realities of nature and that its principles were "responsive to nature's vested and unimpeachable goal: namely, that woman, the nurturant, be her womanly self." For this reason, he was certain that the League would "outlast" feminism.[28] It is important to note that neither Ratner nor League ideology is concerned at all that naming mothering as woman's "natural" role has a history of exploitation and oppression. Within the context of this study, however, I believe it more to the point to note that Ratner's statement demonstrates a lack of understanding of the full scope of feminism as well as a less-than-complete understanding of the organization that was so close to his heart.

From the organization's inception, the women of La Leche League have been as influenced as other women by the changes and dilemmas that have confronted them in the latter half of the twentieth century. Some of these dilemmas they have held in common only with the women of their immediate culture, but regarding the issue that most concerned them, the decline of breast feeding, they encountered a crisis shared by women all over the world. Like the women who are more self-aware of their feminism, when La Leche League members recognized a need for change, they determined to implement it.

La Leche League's faith that women can change the direction of a culture has extended beyond the help offered to individual mothers. League leaders work unceasingly to bring their concepts to the attention of the wider community. From its shoestring, unorganized beginnings to a worldwide organization with a clear philosophy and the respect of several medical associations, as well as the World Health Organization, La Leche League has been persistent in its efforts to influence the medical community through physicians' seminars and similar workshops for other medical personnel. These efforts have often been well rewarded.

CONVERTING MEDICAL PROFESSIONALS

When La Leche League was founded in 1956, there existed several major areas of difference between League concepts about infant care and those of the prevailing medical experts of the time. Since then, however, two of the League's most central concepts — "breast milk is the superior infant food" and "for the healthy, full-term baby, breast milk is the only food necessary until baby shows signs of needing solids (about the middle of the first year of life)" — have come to be accepted by the majority of health care professionals. The American Academy of Pediatrics and the Canadian Paediatric Society made a joint statement in 1979 that strongly recommended breast feeding. The statement expressed a firm belief that human milk was superior to formula. Although the document stressed the importance of breast feeding in those parts of the world where the means for sanitizing water and bottles for formula feeding are inadequate, it also reported that even in areas that enjoy a high standard of living, "less illness is reported among breastfed babies than among bottle-fed infants."[29] Several other national pediatric societies followed suit, and in 1979 the World Health Organization issued a statement in Geneva that read, "Breastfeeding is an integral part of the reproduction process, the natural and ideal way of feeding the infant, and a unique biological and emotional basis for child development."[30]

To find themselves supported by these associations was a potent source of encouragement for the League. The original and more dynamic source of strength, however, was the La Leche League leaders' firm faith that, as women and as breast-feeding mothers, they had knowledge and abilities physicians lacked. They refused to accept the prevalent, scientific "way of knowing." Although women's "ways of knowing" had been gradually discredited with the rise of scientific medicine, the founding mothers and their followers confidently rebelled against the control of knowledge by the predominately male medical world. Such confidence was necessary in an era when the field of infant nutrition belonged to the "experts" and not to the parents of the child. The patriarchal world that was medicine at the turn of the century had become powerful by "cornering the market," so to speak, on knowledge about well-baby care. To speak against such a powerful majority required both courage and diplomacy. One leader, Betty Harris, related that she "came out of the closet and exposed myself as a La Leche League leader" to her children's pediatrician. She told him that she would like to have him understand her approach in helping women who want to breast-feed their babies. He was very willing to set up an appointment because he believed that contact with La Leche League made many women in his practice feel guilty. Clearly, he perceived himself as a savior of women from the League radicals. This perception is often encountered by feminists in other endeavors. The doctor and the leader talked for an entire hour, an unheard of concession on the part of a "busy professional" when dealing with a "mere mother." She explained the La Leche League approach that begins with trying to find out what the mother really wants to do, tells mothers how to accomplish their own goals, and, finally, gives them some alternatives to consider. The doctor had clearly expected that Harris, who was not a medical professional, was giving out dangerous advice and seemed quite relieved to hear about her approach.

Their conversation went on to cover several areas in which mothers might need help. In the end, the doctor admitted that the leader knew a great deal more about nursing than he did and that the League obviously suffered from bad press. The doctor promised to refer patients needing help with breast feeding to her.[31]

This was not an isolated incident. During the late 1970s many doctors and other health care professionals began to promote breast feeding actively. Many of them sent mothers interested in breast feeding to La Leche League for information and support they felt unprepared to give. Information alone, they recognized, could not compare with advice and support given in an atmosphere of personal mother-to-mother reassurance.

From the vantage point of almost forty years, the founding mothers' belief that they could make a difference appears to have been justified. As the League has engaged in cooperation with and opposition to the mainstream medical community, it has been influential in stimulating an alternative perspective on infant nutrition. Still, the dilemma continues of a medical world that strongly recommends breast feeding but often remains unprepared to help when difficulties occur. Women are only marginally recognized as givers of wisdom in the area of well-baby care, which has been absorbed by the medical establishment. Feminists who fight for recognition in the public sphere complain of a "glass ceiling." League women sometimes bump against the glass wall that separates "lay" and "professional" in the medical world.

A WORLDWIDE MISSION

In one central area La Leche League's perspective was ahead of that of many mid-twentieth-century feminists who focused on the liberation of Western middle-class women. By the mid-1960s, the League's outreach beyond middle-class America was well organized. Almost every issue of the *La Leche League News* carried one or more stories about League activities the world over. Leaders demonstrated a sensitivity to the multicultural milieux within which they worked. They asked themselves how the voice of leaders from other cultures could most effectively become a part of League writings and policy. They recognized that changes in administration and communication were necessary because leaders from other countries had different problems and faced different situations.[32]

The following is a dramatic but not necessarily untypical report of the

League's work in the developing areas of the world. Sometimes group meetings or phone counseling is not possible. In 1982, three Guatemalan League leaders were invited by a local pediatrician to make a presentation to the women in the government prison in Guatemala City. (At that time in Guatemala, many incarcerated mothers were allowed to keep their children with them until the children were seven years old.) The women in this prison were ministered to by nuns of the Good Shepherd order. Thus, their quarters were well cared for. Because of these conditions and because the mothers were with their children all but four hours of the day, the leaders felt breast-feeding counseling could succeed. The questions raised by the incarcerated mothers were the same ones League mothers heard wherever they went. The jailed mothers were as hungry for mother-to-mother advice as were mothers outside the prison. Even though some of the mothers were murderers and drug smugglers, the leaders experienced none of the harassment, shouting, or bad language a doctor had warned them to expect. As the leaders continued their work with these mothers, they were called on to solve many of the same difficulties earlier mothers had brought to the founding mothers. For instance, the women in charge of the prison nursery accused the imprisoned women of spoiling their babies if they nursed on demand. Also, nursing babies had been given bottles, so their mothers were having difficulty maintaining their milk supply. Just as at any League meeting, while the leaders talked and listened, their own infants nursed and crawled about at their feet. The leaders noticed one striking difference between these prison "meetings" and those they had led at home: "We've never seen such quick action on our suggestions before!"[33]

LA LECHE FATHERHOOD:
A UNIQUE APPROACH

La Leche League founders realized from the beginning of the movement that attempts to change society without first effecting changes within the family were apt to fail. Whereas they have stressed that any concept of equality must realistically take into account differing abilities and aptitudes and have believed that parental roles are not interchangeable, they find other role divisions arbitrary and unnecessarily restrictive. The earliest edition of the manual urged a rethinking of the traditional division of roles within family life. It argued against the prevailing ideology,

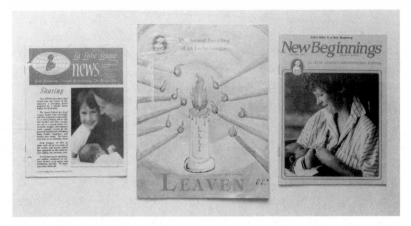

Beginning in 1958, the League began to publish a newsletter. At first called *La Leche League News*, its title was later changed to *New Beginnings*. The League also publishes a newsletter for leaders, *Leaven*. These publications are filled with narratives that testify to the importance of woman-to-woman networking.

which ruled that certain actions such as child care or household chores were "woman's work" and that any man who valued his masculinity should avoid them at all costs. It was far more important, from a League viewpoint, to consider who a father *is* within the family than what he *does* when at home.

Later editions of the manual and subsequent newsletters continued to express a nontraditional understanding of the father's role within the home. Even though most League families followed the traditional divisions of father as provider and mother as nurturer, League fathers were uncommonly concerned with child-care issues. The League's original newsletter, the *La Leche League News*, devoted one issue a year solely to fathers. In 1985, the League changed the format of this publication to a journal, *New Beginnings*, which has carried a regular section entitled "Focus on Fathers," creating a forum for the letters that fathers wrote to the editors, sharing their experiences and requesting information. These letters reveal men who do a great deal of reading on the subject of child care to learn everything they possibly can on the subject.

Still, the League approach is problematic from a liberal feminist point of view. For League mothers this interest in infant care is an outgrowth of the father's unique role in the family. League ideology holds strongly to the ideal of complementary maternal and paternal roles. It understands a child as relating strongly to one parent at certain moments in her life, while at other times in her life the other parent is better able to meet her needs. According to League theory, fathers cannot be perceived as an addendum to the mothering role. Like the mother, the father is "a body for baby to feel and explore, a mind to discover, and a person to share a unique relationship with." The role of the father evolves from infancy forward, a role that grows and changes just as the mother-child relationship does. Mothers and fathers are both understood to be strong nurturers but not as providing the same kind of nurturing.[34] This approach contains some of contemporary feminism's new realism about motherhood and fatherhood. League mothers have long demanded a more active participation by fathers in infant and child care.

Here, one cannot help but note that, although the women of La Leche League may live out many feminist precepts, the League's ideology completely ignores a long-standing feminist critique. As Simone de Beauvoir points out in *The Second Sex*, women have always been defined by men. This includes not only defining their place in society as secondary but also naming the way women's biology designates this place. League ideology makes no attempt to break away from the assumption that biology defines child-care roles. The actions of the women of La Leche League, however, manifest a rejection of traditional boundaries in other areas of domestic responsibility and a nontraditional willingness to take a public role customarily prescribed for women. The League has also sought through meetings, conferences, professional seminars, and literature to change society's values regarding the institutions of family and work.

NETWORKING TO MAKE A DIFFERENCE

One important source of La Leche League's ability to offer and effect these important changes in the private and the public sphere is women's socialized ability to network with other women to the benefit of all within the network. In Carol Gilligan's study on the moral development of women, *In a Different Voice*, feminine perceptions of reality are shown to be based on a socialization process that differs radically from that of men. Gilligan found that there exist in our culture "two modes of describing the relationship between other and self." Women's ways of seeing the world are distinctive, and consequently women base their decisions for acting on different premises than men do. Gilligan believes differentiating influences enter the child's earliest years and are constantly reinforced. How her mother sees her own role in society and the fact that the adult community expects the daughter to hold herself to these patterns are two realities perceived by the female child even before she acquires language. Gilligan concludes that in Western culture, "masculinity is defined through separation while femininity is defined through attachment." Some aspects of these gender-based lines of development can be limiting for men and especially for women. More positively, however, women reach adulthood with a strong sense of responsibility to their community and a belief in the importance of intimacy, relationships, and care.[35]

Women act on the basis of these principles to help one another. Feminists have networked in innumerable directions to end the oppressive limits to the culture's roles for women. La Leche League women network to help women who wish to breast-feed fulfill this dream whatever their circumstances.

A woman-to-woman connection is unquestionably necessary to create the trusting situation in which the League perspective can flourish and the dominant culture can be transformed. This can be true even for a woman well schooled about breast feeding. Flor Constantino belonged to La Leche League for nine years. This was a time of gradually escalating involvement that led to her becoming assistant area coordinator of leader applicants. When in the spring of 1984 she became isolated from the League because she had moved to a remote area of Oregon, she had a discouraging round of correspondence with the League's international headquarters and began to question whether to continue her work. Later, however, the traumatic experience of giving birth to her son two and a half months prematurely brought her back to the League. Because her son Nicholas was born in a hospital 130 miles away from Flor's home, she came into contact with the League leader in that city.

That leader, Jan LaChapelle, assisted the Constantinos through the many harrowing moments of the fight for their son's survival. She was their best advocate at the hospital and in the community. Her assistance included visiting their son Nicholas when they could not make the long trip to the hospital. Finally, after two months, Flor Constantino was allowed to bring home her tiny infant, who weighed only three pounds nine ounces. The doctor stated that her experience as a La Leche League leader made him confident that she would be able to handle Nicholas's special care.[36]

The Constantinos' story is just one of many in League literature demonstrating that the woman-to-woman connection has been a major source of La Leche League's strength. Two studies conducted in the 1970s demonstrate the importance of this woman-to-woman support. The first was based on the deductions psychologist Alice Ladas accumulated from a 1970 survey given to 1,124 pregnant women who planned to breast-feed and who originally came to La Leche League for information. Ladas wished to establish to what extent information and support are correlated with the outcome of breast feeding. In particular, Ladas hoped to answer whether there was some instinctual reason that contemporary women were so unsuccessful at breast feeding or whether it was simply the lack of support that accounted for this phenomenon. For the women who continued to attend meetings or to keep in touch with the leader, the study confirmed Ladas's hypothesis that neither information nor support alone was as beneficial as the combination of information with human support. She discovered that her figures also supported the findings of Solomon Asch that if informed support for an endeavor is present, the existence of individuals who dispute the choice does not seriously modify behavior.

Of the 756 mothers in the group who did not continue breast feeding, 31 percent chose to stop because of early difficulties such as sore nipples, insufficient milk, or poor sucking by the baby. Because of intervention by doctors, nurses, or other hospital personnel, fully 20 percent discontinued breast feeding before they themselves wanted to stop. Ladas believed her findings justified a call for the retraining of hospital personnel so that they could help mothers wishing to breast-feed. She also acknowledged, however, that, although beginning well in the hospital is important, belonging to a supportive group of mothers after the hospital stay was the best insurance that a good start would become a successful endeavor. Those mothers in the study who continued to breast-feed were the ones who received information as well as both individual and group support.[37]

In 1976, Hannah Meara published the results of sociological research that studied the League's particular approach to breast-feeding counseling. Meara was concerned that, though breast feeding had been proven to be beneficial to infant, mother, and community, the rate of breast feeding continued to decline. This, she noted, was true even though in the United States women with high levels of formal education were increasingly initiating breast feeding. These women wished to nurse their babies, but many of them were not able to establish a successful breast-feeding pattern. When they encountered the ensuing frustration, the women discovered that they lived in a society where bottles, not breasts, were the endorsed and fitting vessels and conveyors of a baby's nourishment. Meara noted that these women resided where medical personnel frequently extend disheartening, conflicting, and even harmful advice. Some mothers, she found, turned to La Leche League for advice and support. These mothers, it seemed, were more successful. In order to determine why this was the case, Meara gathered information about League methods by observing participants at League meetings, conducting in-depth interviews with mothers, and administering a national survey. For comparison, she and her team interviewed obstetrical nurses and breast-feeding mothers who were not affiliated with the League.[38]

Her research revealed that, for the latter group, breast feeding was understood to be a more limited experience than it was for women affiliated with La Leche League. The report examined each of those perspectives that Meara held to be central to the League's philosophy and support patterns.[39] The study demonstrated that League women were not bound by a compatibility of any previously held individual viewpoints but instead shared the experience of having assimilated new ways. Meara discovered the same pattern for each League perspective: affiliated mothers handled the various crises of breast feeding bolstered by techniques and convictions learned through the League, whereas unaffiliated mothers often gave in to pressures from medical doctors and others to give up nursing.

League perspectives on hospital routines, nursing schedules, and, later, weaning frequently placed the League in conflict with physicians and other health care personnel. In the face of these obstacles, the mothers affiliated with the League were more likely than unaffiliated mothers to persist, because of the strength and collective character of the League perspective. For example, the team observed that at group meetings, characteristically, babies who cried were nursed immediately. New mothers who offered pacifiers or made other distractive maneuvers were gently persuaded to nurse the baby instead.

This example is significant because both undernourished breast-fed infants and understimulated lactation mechanisms commonly cause serious problems for American breast-feeding couples. Meara discovered that usually the unaffiliated mother's perspective was that a three-to-four-and-a-half-hour schedule was good for themselves and for their babies. La Leche League members, on the other hand, were unconcerned about the timings of feedings. Instead, they focused on responding to the baby's expression of need.

Another distinctive perspective studied was the concept routinely upheld by League mothers of the late introduction of solid food. These mothers introduced solids at four to six months. This contrasted with giving solids between six to eight weeks, the time frame customarily prescribed by American physicians. This practice differed sharply from that of unaffiliated mothers, who did not connect the introduction of solids with breast feeding. Their goal in introducing solids, usually when the baby was around one month old, was to ensure that the baby would sleep through the night. They made this decision on the basis of their doctor's advice or information garnered from baby books.

Meara concluded that, for many League mothers, La Leche League is a way of life. For these women, the League way provides solutions to breast feeding and related problems that women encounter in mothering young infants.

Meara found it remarkable that the League had socialized mothers to group outlooks that the prevailing culture did not support. It demonstrated, she believed, the importance of emotional, as well as informational, support from others with similar experiences. She discovered that no matter how willing or well meaning a male doctor or a husband might be, he cannot give the support that comes from having similar experiences. It takes, Meara contended, other women to do so. She pointed out that in a breast-feeding culture this happens naturally but in a bottle-feeding culture an organization like the League becomes necessary.

Meara acknowledged that League members were vociferous in their advocacy. (Similar attacks are made on feminists.) In their defense, though, Meara wrote that the reason League members were often seen as fanatical was that "countering the cultural mainstream is an arduous task. . . . Once they are mobilized for this essential and difficult battle, it may be difficult for them to see amidst the fray the difference between readily solvable problems and the essentially unsolvable psychological and/or physiological problems which a small minority of mothers encounter."[40]

La Leche League mothers are not some group apart from women with feminist concerns. Their lament is like that of Bonnie Miller-McLemore: "I am neither inside nor wholly outside the traditions and cultures that have held me and those that have liberated me."[41] In the League, women find a community to which they can belong. It is a community with its own traditions and rituals. It also has its own wisdom that accepts the tenets of science but grounds them in a religious dimension. This dimension is expressed in an explicit faith in the healing support of a women's network. It can also be discovered in the League's implicit acceptance of a family theology found in many religious traditions but best known to the founding mothers through their upbringing in and continued alliance with the American Roman Catholic Church.

chapter 6

· ·

The Evolution of a Catholic Theology of the Family

THE IMPACT OF THE FAITH DIMENSION
ON LA LECHE LEAGUE

The League sees its members as a powerful force within both the private and the public sphere, and it stresses that their strength and their insights are rooted in motherhood. The League's answer to the question "What should mothers do?" is, however, grounded in the correlation between its praxis and that of the original faith community of its founders.[1]

For those women, the contents of their Catholic faith and the existential questions of motherhood are interdependent. Their understanding of the nature of their universe, not only its scientific facts and its human relationships but also its determinative context, shaped their answers to every question they faced. Just as concepts from the biological and the human sciences help to construct reality for League members, so do those concepts garnered from the sacred dimension of their lives. While all three sources contribute to the League's religious way of being in the world, the tenets of the faith community of the founders, the American Catholic Church, are the least acknowledged. Approaching League

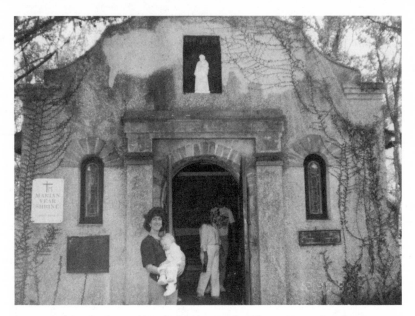

Maria Hidalgo Dolan and her fourteen-month-old son Alexander visit the shrine of Our Lady of La Leche in St. Augustine, Florida, in December 1989.

praxis through an understanding of its parallels with Catholicism requires a distinction between the "sense" (or deep meaning) and the "referents" (the sources) of its texts.[2] The "referents" of the League texts are its medical, sociological, and psychological perceptions. Clarifying the "sense" of its texts requires an examination of the League's social context. An exploration of the Catholic way of being in the world as it relates to the norms developed by the League to guide mothers and fathers in the care of their children demonstrates that these norms are grounded not simply in theories about good parenting but "in the concrete intellectual, moral and religious praxis of concrete human beings in distinct societal and historical situations."[3]

Because the founders of La Leche League were Catholic, there exist strong parallels between the basic concepts and practices of La Leche League and Catholic family theology in mid-twentieth-century America. Theologians of culture have noted that the values of even the most secular persons are actually religious values that have become part of the culture, and feminist theologians further claim that women who have undergone religious education are doubly socialized into their cultural roles. Anthropologists and other social scientists have demonstrated that cultural factors affect a woman's sense of herself. Therefore, in answering questions of ultimate meaning, La Leche League, born in the 1950s in America, inevitably drew on the metaphorical language of its culture. This culture was immersed in the metaphors of a Western religious heritage. In addition, all the founders of the League were Catholic. From the time the founders were children until they were new mothers, the basic beliefs of their faith community were grounded in papal teachings seldom questioned by laypersons. From the time of Pope Leo XIII through the end of the twentieth century, family issues have received significant attention. Papal teaching of this era cohered around a "theologically inspired emphasis on divine and human unity yielding a cluster of shared insights on human relations in society. These insights are dicrotic, or double-pulsed, in that, they entail both positive recommendations and negative judgments regarding the general concepts of God, humanity, and the world, and specific practices and ideas touching religious, political, family, economic, and cultural life."[4]

These recommendations and judgments were not taken without questioning. In fact, they were held in a dialectical relationship to the practices of Catholic life. As founder Mary White states, "It isn't that Catholics read the encyclicals in order to know what to believe and how to act. It's that the encyclicals reflect what most Catholics already believe and the way most Catholics are already acting." Similarly, Donald R. Campion, a leading Catholic sociologist, holds that the most characteristic achievement of Vatican II was a synthesis of Catholic thinking on social issues. He believes that most Catholics already believed most teachings set forth by the council.[5]

I do not claim that La Leche League is Catholic. It is not. Certain correspondences to Catholicism, however, illustrate that the League held a religious rather than a secular view of the family. Despite its reliance on the science of infant nutrition and the politics of women's networks, at a deep level the League philosophy relied on metaphors familiar since childhood to reveal its perception of the world. "We used to read and reread *Child and Family Digest,*" according to Marian Tompson. "It supported the way we were inclined and was a good education for all of us."[6]

Three central concepts within the Roman Catholic perspective parallel La Leche League theories. Both organizations understand biology to be the foundation for moral obligation. Both perceive love as service to others but not as self-sacrifice. And both practice evangelization through role modeling rather than active proselytizing. Each of these concepts was uniquely expressed in the American Catholic context, the culture of the founders. Although an evolution in the interpretation of each concept has occurred during the latter half of this century, their core validity is still accepted by both the League and many members of the American Catholic faith community.

THE AMERICAN CATHOLIC FAMILY
IN THE MID-TWENTIETH CENTURY

The American Catholic family of the mid-twentieth century was no longer the immigrant or newly naturalized Catholic family of the early part of the century. Most American Catholics had assimilated the patterns of life common to middle- and working-class citizens. Within American Catholic families, however, the movement from practice to theory to reformed practice differs in three important ways from that of other Western faith communities. First, Catholic moral discernment is grounded in a particular understanding of natural law theory.[7] Second, Catholics understand that the family, not the individual, is the essential cell of human society. In addition, the family serves as a haven of love not only for its members but also for all community members in need. Within these Catholic families, the understanding of love focuses on interdependence, downplaying self-sacrifice. Mary, the mother of Jesus, as a model of this kind of love, is the object of a distinctive Catholic piety. Third, for Catholics, marriage is a sacrament. It is a sign to the community of Christ's presence among them.

NATURAL LAW THEORY: SOURCE OF
AMBIGUITY AND SECURITY

The belief that there exists a natural law that serves as a divine guide for human morality has been a source of both ambiguity and security for American Catholics. The ambiguity is rooted in the enigmatic elements in Thomas Aquinas's concept of natural law, elements that appear in the League's understanding of right and wrong ways to parent. Aquinas's concept of natural law wavers between the order of nature and the order of reason. His general thrust is toward the primacy of reason in natural law theory, although his writings include certain tendencies to identify the requirements of natural law with physical and biological processes.

Like Aristotle before him and Aquinas's own later interpreters, Aquinas relied on a contemporary understanding of the human situation. His understanding of the role of women in society reflected his perception of their bodily reality. Thus, as Lisa Cahill observes, "He makes a good example both of the necessary dependence of the theologian on contributory disciplines, and of the peril of placing too serene a confidence in the conclusions of these other sciences."[8]

Papal teachings reiterated late scholastic formulas for natural law. For Pope Leo XIII, the law of nature was the same as the eternal reason of God.[9] Pius XI insisted that because human nature is rooted in God, human rights are inextricably linked with divinely mandated duties to God, self, and neighbor.[10] In contrast, moral theologian Henry Davis emphasized that natural law is biological but is discerned by reason. For Davis, the precepts of natural law resulted from our ability to apprehend certain natural inclinations as being good. He contended that because natural appetites are the same in all humans, the first principles of natural law were universal; however, since everyone's life and circumstances are not the same, natural law does not exact the same obligations from everyone everywhere.[11]

The Second Vatican Council ratified no specific directives for moral theology. It conducted no inquiry into the adequacy of natural law theory as a basis for Catholic moral directives. Instead, the bishops called on all Catholics, not just clergy, to develop a moral theology that would increase the fruits of love in the world. Thus, despite its ambiguity, natural law thinking remained the anchor for Roman Catholic moral theology in the mid-twentieth century.

THE CATHOLIC FAMILY: HAVEN OF LOVE

The Catholic Church in the post-Leonine period has asserted that the family, as the essential cell of human society, is both haven of love for its members and light to the world.[12] Throughout this period, popes have stressed that Christian families are the foundation of the social society. John XXIII warned that, should Christian marriage falter, the foundations of the nation would tremble. He asked, "Unless peace, unity, and concord are present in domestic society, how can they exist in civil soci-

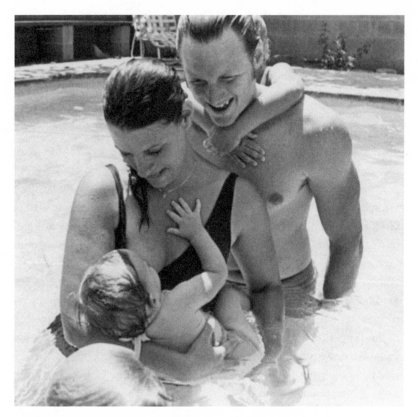

The family as the central unit of society is a focus shared by Catholicism and La Leche League. Here Debbie and Jack Bray of Saugus, California, enjoy family time with Stacy (on Dad's back), Christy (nursing), and Chad (foreground).

ety?"[13] The twentieth-century popes have offered a consistent portrait of the ideal family. In such a family, parents are abundantly loving, children are numerous, and all are industrious and religious. Family members are compassionate and share what they have with the poor. Papal teaching depicts family life as rooted in monogamous marriage. Partners are perpetually bound by love and the sanctity of their union. These principles are grounded in Catholic scriptural theology and are held to have existed from the creation of the human race.

Recent encyclicals have also emphasized that parents are the natural caregivers and educators of their children. Any force that wrests this charge away from them is considered a violation of parental rights. Family and nation each have differentiated rights. It is vital that the state not intrude on the mission given by God to parents. This mission is balanced between the obligation to create a haven of love for one another and their children and the call to reflect to the world God's presence within it.

For Catholics marriage is a sacrament precisely because Christ perfected it by rendering the couple's natural love spiritual as well. As a haven from the world, the family is expected to exhibit an intense caring for one another and a joyous acceptance of God's will. Pius XII envisioned this spiritualized family as one without "the turmoil of quarreling or the agony of infidelity where children are perceived pledges of God's love and the love of the couple for one another. Thus, no material motive frustrates the gift of life." Exemplary Catholic parents are expected to be as concerned with the spiritual growth and moral well-being of their children as they are with their healthy physical development.[14]

In the mid-twentieth century, pastors and theologians worried that the rapidly occurring changes in American life would cause American Catholics to embrace mainstream values even if they conflicted with Catholic ones. Catholics were urged to develop a strong interdependence within the family as a counterweight to the secularization of the dominant culture. This culture was perceived as encouraging premarital intimacy, sanctioning divorce, and advising birth control. American Catholic families believed themselves distinct from this secular society and strove to strengthen the family against its intrusions. Despite ethnic, social, political, and regional diversities, Catholics developed a group consciousness that lead to considerable solidarity.

Just how distinctive Catholic family life really was or is from life within other families is debatable. Not the reality but the Catholic ideal of family life, however, was a major motivator of decisions within actual Catholic families. In this ideal four major patterns stand out: the importance of children; a traditional structure, characterized by spouses assuming complementary roles; love of others as love of self; and devotion to Mary.

CHILDREN: THE CENTER OF MARRIED LIFE

First and foremost, official Catholic teaching and popular Catholic practice upheld the concept that children were integral to family life. When couples married, they expected to conceive, care for, and educate children. Notions regarding this principle within Catholicism are often entangled with debates about birth control. Midcentury Catholics were aware that birth control issues set official Catholic teaching apart from that of other religious communities and from the secular society. In the 1940s, 1950s, and early 1960s, individual Catholics did not experience the ambiguity Catholics have endured since 1968.[15] The popes had made it very clear that the church rejected contraception, condemned abortion, and forbade sterilization, and few Catholics openly challenged this stance.

Despite all the public debate birth control has engendered since 1968, this issue is not a focal point within the full scope of Catholic family theology. Church teaching consistently holds that marriage and conjugal love are naturally ordained toward having children. Yet, while the bishops of the Second Vatican Council praised couples who with careful reflection undertook to bring up a large family, they stressed that a large family is not per se the goal. The conception of each child needed to be weighed against the material and spiritual needs of every other member of the family.

HUSBAND AND WIFE:
A COMPLEMENTARY TEAM

Responsible parenthood required an atmosphere of stability and well-being. Within the Western context, this responsibility fell mostly on mothers. Therefore, women's struggle for emancipation produced papal concerns about its negative effects on the solidarity of family life. Some Catholic women themselves expressed this concern. In 1960 in *Women in Wonderland*, Dorothy Dohen declared that in the secular family pattern women marry young, have one or two children immediately, and then return to employment when the youngest child enters grade school. Dohen deplored this paradigm as distorting family life. She praised those Catholic wives who rejected this process, staying faithful to important Catholic values by remaining at home throughout their children's childhood.[16] Ironically, earlier papal injunctions had been directed at both parents equally. A mother's particular biology was not understood to render her more responsible than the father for the care and education of their children. But within the mid-twentieth-century context, with its clear division between the private and the public sphere, this principle was lost.

The family model that is often referred to as "traditional" is actually a social and political construct of the late nineteenth and early twentieth century. Midcentury Catholics, however, perceived this model not as a socially constructed one but as the family pattern designed by God for the good of all humans. Within this pattern husbands and wives had specific, complementary parts to play.

Papal teaching has emphasized that the differences between husbands and wives are not differences of equality. Women were acknowledged as having a right to all the dignities that belong to humans simply by virtue of being human. The authority of husbands could not be used to deny wives their liberty. Not only did the wife have the right to refuse any request of her husband's that was not reasonable, but she had the responsibility to assume authority in the household if her husband neglected his obligations to his family. The popes did assume that a certain inequality would result from accommodations that spouses agreed to for the stability of family life. Wives were exhorted to accept husbands' decisions with which they disagreed in order to maintain family harmony. The popes did, however, insist that such accommodations should neither compromise the loving nature of the marital relationship nor trample on consensual rights due to all persons as human beings. Dohen held that both scriptural and encyclical statements on Christian subjection of wife to husband allowed for considerable latitude. Those who interpreted the Christian texts as rigorously demanding a definite set of rules based such interpretations more on cultural values than any Catholic strictures.[17] Nevertheless, some Catholic thought reveals a perception of the complementarity of husbands and wives as a natural difference that fits men and women to play different roles within family life.

In the *Summa Theologiae*, Aquinas reiterates Aristotle's concept of women as misbegotten males. Furthermore, Aquinas suggests that, except in the area of generation, men find better helpmates in other men than they do in women.[18] Although notions of innate differences between male and female nature did become a part of Catholic understanding, this Aquinian speculation on the nature of women never became a part of Catholic doctrine. Instead, various positions on the nature of men and women evolved along the lines of equal but different. The traditional and official position contended that biological differences between men and women were the sources of differences in temperament as well as abilities. The encyclicals also conveyed the belief that natural differences required that women be protected in schools and in the workplace. Leo XIII was convinced that women were unsuited for certain occupations outside the home. In fact, he claimed that women were naturally fitted for housework.[19] Such a contention seems laughable when one considers the hard labor involved in housework in Leo's time. What is clearly at work here is an assumption that women must be protected not from hard labor but from unnecessary exposure to an evil world.

An alternative position offered in the 1960s accepted natural biological differences while rejecting the idea that personality differences are a natural result of sexual differences. Proponents of this theory acknowledged that, biologically, women are made for motherhood and men are made for fatherhood, but they emphasized that this fact does not magically render women more compassionate, more sympathetic, more emotional, or more moral. Dissimilarities in sex roles evolve under the influence of culture. Personality differentiation happens in a milieu of societal expectations. In reality, women differ more extensively among themselves then they differ as a group compared to men.[20]

A third theme was articulated by Catholic feminist theologian Katherine Zappone in 1991. This position holds that biology endows women with an essential feminine character so that they are better equipped for the nurturing roles of motherhood. This position resembled the traditional Catholic stance but diverged from it by calling for a radical shift in the "cultural valuing of mothering." For Zappone, identifying the innate womanly characteristics would clarify the sex-specific contributions women have to offer in the public domain.[21]

What women might offer in the public sphere was seldom the subject of Catholic teaching, until very recently. Most Catholic thinking on male-female complementarity, as expressed through the teachings of its hierarchy and the practices of its families, centered on a concern for the overall welfare of the family. Many of the popes worried that families would suffer if women sought freedom from the duties of spouse and mother by entering into business and public affairs. They were also concerned that economic freedom for women would weaken women's acceptance of the responsibility for family nurture.

Three aspects of the notion of complementarity appear in Catholic literature: concerns about women in the workplace; specific roles for men and women; and a wife's subordination to her husband. The three aspects intertwine to form a consistent policy.

From the late nineteenth through the mid-twentieth centuries, the Catholic Church consistently opposed the presence of women in the workplace. Pius XI maintained the position that the employment of any woman, but especially the employment of wives, encouraged the neglect of all family duties, most especially the rearing of children. His position was widely embraced by the American Catholics throughout most of this century. Before the second wave of feminism began in the 1960s, the most prominent exception to the total domestication of women was the labor shortage that occurred during World War II. This shortage led to a national reevaluating of the necessity for wives and mothers to remain housebound. Despite this secular transformation, the American Catholic hierarchy resisted any change in women's status. The church believed that allowing women to work in the war effort would endanger religious values. Bishop John Duffy of Buffalo claimed that, if women went to work, the sanctity of the home would be lost. This loss would then threaten the nation's ability to win the war. On another front, Bishop John O'Hara of Philadelphia condemned the Women's Auxiliary Army Corps because it ignored the duties allocated to women and threatened the inviolability of the family. Church officials and many Catholic writers worried that women would not readily give up their jobs when the war was over. They were concerned that, far from being a step toward equality, employment outside the home would destroy women's natural dignity. When the war ended, the bishops warned that if women did not return to their divinely ordained mission of homemaker, peace could not last. As the postwar era blended into the early 1950s, the nation as a whole accepted that wives and mothers should not be employed outside the home, but it was American Catholic writers and churchmen who were in the vanguard of this movement. In 1951, Cardinal Cushing of Boston forthrightly declared that it was not Catholic for women to work after marriage.[22]

Although post–Vatican II encyclicals contained no specific criticism of the women's emancipation movement, papal encyclicals after the council continued to view as problematic any situation that necessitated the mother's working outside the home. Employment of mothers, it was feared, endangered the established roles of men and women within the family. Men were expected to be wage earners and heads of household, and women were to administer to the daily wants and needs of the household. In accordance with earlier papal teachings, John XXIII taught that the household at Nazareth provided the model for the Christian family. This role division was considered essential to the success of marriage and family life. Although it recognized that husbands and wives carried the major responsibility for assuming their "appropriate" roles, the church also called on society as a whole and the couple's immediate community to support husbands and wives in maintaining this family structure. Both Pius XI and Pius XII bade government and business to ensure that all fathers of families received a just wage, which was defined as one sufficient to support both the worker and his family.

Until the late 1970s, Catholic teaching held that the husband was the ultimate authority in the marital relationship. This understanding was based on theology rooted in a particular view of the relationship of the church and Christ. Leo XIII wrote, "Since the husband represents Christ, and since the wife represents the Church, let there always be, both in him who commands and in her who obeys, a heaven-born love guiding both in their respective duties."[23] Leo saw the husband as the ruler of the family and the head of the family. For him, the wife was expected to obey her husband. This was not, Leo claimed, the obedience of a servant. Rather, it was the honorable and dignified obedience of a companion. This distinction is one that is hard to uphold. Companions are generally regarded as equals and their relationship as grounded in dialogue, not in the obedience of one to the other. Yet John XXIII would sustain this teaching, naming the husband as the ultimate authority in the family and continuing to insist that a wife's "primary role" was to submit to that authority. Recent scholarship has questioned the fidelity of this interpretation to biblical entreaty, and feminists have demonstrated its destructiveness within the marital relationship.

Such teachings were, however, readily accepted by mid-twentieth-century Catholics. Although many Catholic women continued working after marriage, they perceived their husbands as the preferred family providers. If it was possible, they most often thankfully retired from outside employment as soon as possible after becoming pregnant. The mid-twentieth-century church community actively promoted the ideal that the mother was responsible for household administration. An ironic twist to this support is revealed in the actions of Winifred C. Stanley of

New York, the first Catholic congresswoman. In 1943, she vigorously endorsed the equal rights amendment that had been first introduced in 1923. At the same time, she claimed that homemaking was a woman's greatest career. Stanley was joined by some other Catholic women in support of the amendment, but most Catholics strongly opposed it. Many individual parishes sanctified these norms by offering a Sunday morning seven o'clock Mass, referred to as "the women's Mass" because it was timed to allow women to return home, complete housework, and start dinner.[24]

Dohen maintained that delegating household tasks to women and wage earning to men could establish a stable pattern in family life. She, however, rejected absolute complementarity by insisting that household chores were in no "essential way" women's work. She noted that parents themselves often arrived at the obvious conclusion that both must contribute at home. Despite her rejection of absolute complementarity, Dohen writes, "Marriage is indeed the way to sanctity. Woman made for man finds in man her way to God."[25] Dohen's observations are intriguing because they reveal the way some women walked the thin line between countering official Catholic positions and supporting an ideal that would threaten their full humanity. Such reflections were the first stirring of religious feminism.

Paul VI broke somewhat with this tradition. In *Populorium Progressio*, he criticized oppressive family structures. He noted that traditional understandings of power between husbands and wives had contributed to historical oppression and even recognized that, within some Catholic families, Pius XI's counsel that headship must always be conducted in total love had been ignored, resulting in sexual oppression. Still, Paul's stance was less a rejection of the principle of the headship of the father than a demand that the father exercise his authority lovingly and without denying the rights of other family members.

LOVING ONE'S PARTNER AS
ONE LOVES ONESELF

Without abandoning the importance of children to family life, from the end of the nineteenth through the middle of the twentieth century, the popes gradually gave renewed attention to spousal affection. In *Arcanum*, Leo XIII identified the happiness of the partners as a major goal of marriage. He viewed their happiness as contributing to their ability to fulfill their duties as just and caring citizens. In *Casti Connubii*, Pius XI wrote, "Man and wife help each other day by day in forming and perfecting themselves in the interior life, so that through their partnership in life they may advance ever more and more in virtue, and above all they may grow in true love toward God and their neighbor."[26]

The love the church envisioned was not easy to fulfill. Men and women were expected to subordinate their individual interests to the demands of the marriage. Sacrifice was a necessary component of married love for both husband and wife. Contemporary Catholic ethicist Stephen Pope notes that theologians writing moral guides at that time understood love as the fulfillment of a law. True, tender feelings might contribute to love, but love was essentially an act of the will performed for God's sake.[27]

Since Vatican II, the popes have moved even further toward emphasizing mutual love as the defining quality of family life. Although there remains a focus on procreation and the care and education of children, this focus is set within the goal of conjugal love. Yet confusion still exists over how to reconcile the notion that love is at the center of family life with the authority of a husband over his wife and the specification of spousal roles by gender. For Catholic women, personalizing their church's values within the particularities of their individual context most often means that as wife and mother they sacrifice their own needs and desires. The demands of modern family life limit opportunities for the mutual love urged by church teachings. Dohen sagely noted that married women seem to have a "mysterious vocation to suffering" and that they are asked to bear, "not their fair share—but their share with Christ, of the sins of the world."[28]

At the same time, however, while Catholic teaching often seems to interpret love as the sacrifice of the self for the sake of others, self-sacrifice is not its true focus. According to traditional Catholic doctrine, charity, or love, is a theological virtue that God confers on humans so that they might love him. The love of others is one of a myriad of opportunities for loving God. Like any virtue, Christian loving is a balance between extremes. Although no one can love God too much, the ways we choose for expressing that love through our love of others must be guided by the Aristotelian mean between extremes.[29] To love others at the exclusion of loving ourselves is such an extreme. Because God's charity will always outreach ours, the example of Christ's sacrifice is only a call for humans to love God to their full capacity. It is not a demand that the Christian sacrifice herself for the sake of others.

Humans speak about the good in ways that have a distinctively premoral sense, that is, we see objects or experiences as good to pursue because they appear enjoyable, valuable, or worthy to promote. "Premoral goods are in themselves neither moral nor immoral, although they can become organized so as to become either."[30] Thus, every choice is in some way a sacrifice because premoral values and disvalues are so connected that we can seldom achieve a premoral value without allowing the inseparable premoral disvalue. When two people marry and have children, some of their subsequent decisions will be an expression of self-determinative autonomy, individually and together. In addition, though, their decisions are informed by priorities that have become an individual way of thinking and doing that results from their education and established social patterns of behavior and of the sense of moral obligation that determines the roles and tasks of their society.

According to midcentury American Catholic cultural norms, the father's obligation to provide for his family and the mother's responsibility to care for the children were accepted premoral values. Any restrictions this placed on the spouses' autonomy were considered unavoidable. Parents viewed their love as mutual. If women seemed to sacrifice more than men did, it was perceived as a necessary choice, as an option for the lesser premoral disvalue.[31] Often the husband's sacrifices were perceived to be at least as great, since many fathers worked two or three jobs in order to maintain the family's financial well-being so that mothers need not resort to employment outside the home.

While the midcentury American Catholic mother and wife shared with non-Catholic women in her era a life most often defined by her role in the domestic sphere, she shared one aspect with only her Catholic peers. This was the centrality of Mary, the mother of Jesus, in the beliefs and practices of the Catholic Church.

MARY, MOTHER AND MODEL

According to Catholic teaching, Mary is a constant source of renewal to which humans may turn. God has blessed her with the very gifts befitting such a role in human life. Hers is not a passive but an active cooperation with God in the work of human salvation.[32] Mary's role as mediatrix between God and humanity has a long history, and devotion to Mary was quite strong from the mid-nineteenth through the mid-twentieth centuries. In 1846, in contrast with earlier popes whose encyclicals called on the Holy Spirit or on Jesus as Christ for aid in human endeavors, Pius IX held Mary up to Catholics as an intercessor for humanity. Because Mary is both with God always and the mother of all humans, she is humanity's best hope for advocacy before God.[33] Pius XII reiterated Mary's role in human redemption. She is, he told the faithful, the second Eve, sent to undo the work of the original Eve. Mary as agent for all humans, free from all sin and united with Christ, offered her son on Golgotha to God the Father. With the same ardent love she exhibited at Calvary, Mary continues to feed and nourish humans as she cherished and fed the infant Jesus.[34]

Papal and popular confidence continued unabated through the late 1960s. John XXIII urged Catholics to turn with ever greater confidence to Mary, who is the constant refuge of Christians in any adversity.[35] In 1964, *Lumen Gentium*, the *Dogmatic Constitution of the Church*, proclaimed that the earliest Scriptures clearly understand Mary as the Mother of the Redeemer. Thus, the church continues to teach that Mary cares for the brothers and sisters of her son who live in contemporary times. Mary's motherly function neither obscures nor diminishes the mediation of Christ, but rather discloses its power. Many Roman Catholics still believe that Mary's influence with the faithful fosters the union of Christ and his people.[36] Walter Abbott, an early commentator on the Vatican II documents, asserted that the section on Mary represented a skillful compromise between "two tendencies in modern Catholic thought." The bishops upheld Mary's unique connection with Christ the Redeemer without diminishing her place as fully human and, thus, a member of the redeemed.[37]

The notion that Mary could serve as a model for all mothers was a major influence on the daily lives of American Catholic women. In *Ubi Primum*, Pius IX revealed his vision of the ideal mother through his description of Mary as mercifully affectionate, working to protect her children from all grief and tribulation.[38]

In *Lumen Gentium*, the bishops named the unfailing and generous love of parents as a model for all Christian love. They maintained that Mary was a model of virtue for the whole community precisely because her life of maternal love was a fitting example of an apostolic mission.[39] Thus emerges a picture of motherhood as an apostolic mission expressed by unfailing love.

As wives and mothers, Catholics were urged to follow the example of Mary by being subject to their husband. It was pointed out to them that, although Mary was undoubtedly Joseph's superior in wisdom and spirituality, it was Joseph who led the Holy Family. Repeatedly, Mary was hailed as the ideal woman, one who devoted herself to housework, meal preparation, and child care. Family disintegration was blamed on women who did not accept this model.[40] That such a picture is woefully uninformed by knowledge of life in the Hebrew communities in which Mary lived has only been uncovered by recent scholarship.

This socialization for Catholic women began in the home, and education, even at the college level, often did not provide women with an opportunity to challenge the rigidity of this vision. In Catholic colleges for women, motherhood was exalted as women's natural sphere, and Mary was proffered as a young woman's best model. On the other hand, feminist theologian Maria Kassel points out that for women who were oppressed the image of Mary often represented the only honored image of womanhood they knew. It is precisely the archetype of "Mary," the Virgin Mother, that can make us aware of the goal of becoming human: the whole human being grows together out of the contradiction of feminine and masculine, unconscious and conscious, earthly and divine.[41] For those women who did relate to Mary, the model of Mary as mother and homemaker gave dignity to their lifestyle. One woman reported that when she felt marginalized, she reminded herself that "the greatest of all human beings was a housewife." For these women, Mary is "the ultimate woman, who did it all with style and grace, and it was real painful for her." Thus, Catholic women modeled their lives on Mary's because, like her, they saw themselves at the center of a family that was a haven of love.[42]

THE CATHOLIC FAMILY:
A LIGHT TO THE WORLD

This haven, however, was never conceived as an isolated refuge from the world. By midcentury, American Catholic women were, with the church's blessing, beginning to play significant roles in the structure of American life. The apostolate of families was of unique importance for the church and for civil society. Also, Catholicism was gaining ground as part of the mainstream American culture.[43] Catholics began to perceive themselves as journeying with the Holy Spirit to promote the Kingdom of God in the world.

There are two paths whereby Catholics as members of families could take this journey. First, the family served as a model of Christian life. This model began with the fidelity of the spouses. An indissoluble marriage was the core of family life. In addition, Catholic families sought to live a life grounded in biblical principles within society. By their way of life, couples aspired to affirm their place as guardians and educators of their children and to defend the independence of the family. According to *Lumen Gentium*, married couples present to all an example of unfailing and generous love. They build up the brotherhood of charity. They work toward the fruitfulness of the church, and their marriages stand as signs of the love with which Christ loves his church.[44]

The ideal married couple was not only faithful and nurturing; the spouses also served as examples of just living through moderate material acquisition. Even before Vatican II, many American Catholics had embraced the virtue of moderation. These families had accepted the ramifications of rejecting the two-breadwinner family model. Such acceptance combined with two other Catholic precepts, the summons to choose a Catholic education for their children and the ban on birth control, to ensure a frugal lifestyle for such families.[45] Catholic leaders and parents hoped that faithful commitment to economic moderation would set an example for Catholic children. For them, the family served as an apprenticeship for discipleship.

A second facet of the family apostolate was active service to the community. The Vatican II "Decree on the Apostolate of the Laity" identified the family as the church's domestic sanctuary that provided active hospitality, promoted justice, and served those in need. As the second half of the century progressed, papal emphasis shifted from episcopally directed lay action to papal promotion of lay-initiated social action. For Catholic women in families, this involved being active in working for a change in society while maintaining their traditional values.

By the 1940s various associations for Catholic lay action existed in the United States, but one group in particular, the Catholic Family Movement (CFM),[46] clearly influenced the thinking of the founders of La Leche League. All but one of the founders were active members at the time of the League's inception, and CFM understandings of Catholic action can be perceived in the League's strategy for community outreach.

The CFM was developed by a Belgian priest, Joseph Cardijn. Its apostolic technique stressed the reform of society over individual education and formation. The CFM began in several American cities in 1947 as a means of sanctifying the home. It called on mothers to recognize the spirituality of their vocation. The organization, however, soon turned to a focus on social outreach. Formally established in 1949 with a Chicago lawyer and his wife, Pat and Patty Crowley, as leaders, by 1958 it had a membership of thirty thousand couples. The CFM focused then, as it does now, on the relationship between society and the family, a focus that made it unusual among family-life organizations. Radically lay-oriented, it involved its members in issues of social justice. The basic structure of the CFM was developed in the 1940s and retains this form today. As in La Leche League, individual members each belonged to a small group that met regularly to offer guidance and support to one another and to plan social outreach actions for the group. These programs often included aiding needy families within the parish, but they could be as far-reaching as taking part in civil rights actions. Also, like the League, the CFM eventually evolved into a national organization that continues to hold yearly conventions. These meetings, like the small group meetings, are designed both to support member families and to plan social justice actions.

By emphasizing the communal nature of Catholicism, the CFM undercuts the individualism of traditional devotional Catholicism. This makes members more conscious of their responsibility to others, especially the poor and the oppressed. The CFM uses an apostolic technique that stresses the transformation of society through the formula of "observe, judge, and act."[47] This formula is echoed by Kaye Lowman in *The LLLove Story*, when she notes that the founders observed a need and judged themselves able to act on it.

While the CFM approach is one of the most apparent ways early League members transposed Catholic praxis to their organization, parallels exist with the other elements just examined. The relationship between Catholicism and La Leche League is unintended and, therefore, subtle and complex. The story of that relationship reveals that religious ways of thinking and being powerfully affect our everyday life, even when we are unaware of their influence.

chapter 7

· ·

The La Leche League Family
Natural, Loving, and Just

THE NATURAL FAMILY

Early League literature contained a certain unsophisticated dependence on an interpretation of natural law. Natural law theory appeared in La Leche League writings under a particular guise, one that for the League's Catholic founders carried enormous moral weight.[1] By combining a particular understanding of Catholic natural law theory with empirical scientific findings, they developed a theory of the good family based on a romantic faith in a providential Nature and in human instincts.

We perceive this latter conviction in League literature which pictures "Nature" as a personified and divine force, one that designed human biology in such a way that certain biological needs and wants serve as the foundation for making better moral choices. Although the League recognizes that the line between the "right" thing to do and the obligatory choice can be a thin one, accusations that women who choose bottle feeding are "immature" or overly "independent" crept into some early League literature. Also, when the founding mothers met to discuss and clarify their goals and beliefs in 1958, Herbert Ratner challenged them with a quote from a turn-of-the-century book. In *The Nursling*, published in 1907 by Pierre Budin, breast milk is named the food provided by nature for infants. Budin blamed bottle feeding for the high infant mortality rate of his time. He believed that mothers were refusing to nurse their infants because it was not fashionable. To him, this meant such mothers denied their infants the "right" to look to her as the source of their food. They were, he held, condemning their babies to the miseries and dangers of artificial feeding.[2]

For the League, the concept that biological needs can be obligatory centered on the act of breastfeeding but encompassed other aspects of child care as well. This enthusiasm for the "natural" guided the League approach to childbirth. Referring to the first twinge of labor, the founders wrote, "Nature allows no turning back, and what woman, so blessed, would want to? Today your baby will be born!"[3] In the first edition of the League manual, the authors claimed that childbirth was a woman's natural function. To hear her baby's first cry is a "crowning moment of achievement" and the beginning of her "career" as a mother.[4]

For League members breast feeding, like childbirth, was a natural function. It was just as unwomanly to bypass breast feeding in favor of bottle feeding as it would be to bypass childbirth in favor of artificial wombs. The founders believed that, although they might be able to model the "art of breastfeeding," no one could actually teach a woman to be a good mother. "All we or anyone else can do is direct you back to wise Nature's plan."[5] Here, however, as throughout their literature, League mothers made no overt moral claims for breast feeding. The emphasis was on good mothering. The choice to breast-feed did not spontaneously render a woman a good mother. League leaders encountered women who approached breast feeding as a contract. The leaders believed that avoidance of guilt was the primary motive of these mothers. Such mothers, they noted, tended to set specific limits to the amount of time they planned to nurse. "She feels that this discharges her debt to society, to God, to nature, to womanhood."[6] They also affirmed that just as breast feeding alone did not make a good mother, so bottle feeding by no means necessarily meant inadequate mothering. The founders assured mothers who had bottle-fed previous babies that they need not feel "guilty" about decisions made out of ignorance, because most important was the love they gave their infants. They felt confident that once mothers learned to breast-feed, they would not want to settle for anything less than the natural way to nourish their infants.

Despite sincere attempts to put aside obligatory language in their advice, many passages about nature in League literature failed to avoid a moral tone. In this literature, "Nature" itself exemplified the ideal nurturer of human mothers. Nursing was perceived as "Nature's way" of helping mothers relax and rest. This personification of nature suggests that the term was employed, probably unconsciously, as a substitute for God language. Like other divine images, Nature had many caring faces. She was teacher as well as mother. "Breastfeeding your baby is the right and proper thing to do and what better time for your children to learn the natural way of doing things."[7] Mary Ann Cahill saw Providence at work in the teaching of breast feeding to other mothers. Her advice disclosed a more Thomistic than Romantic understanding. She perceived an interplay of reason and natural moral instincts in mother-to-mother guidance. She stressed that God structured the human community so that information about mothering would be passed by one generation of women to the next as an opportunity for growth for both mentor and new mother.[8]

League members saw "Nature" working to assure family well-being in many areas, including birth control. The first edition of the manual interpreted the fact that breast feeding affords a natural spacing of children as part of Nature's plan for humanity. Breast feeding, the founders held, because it was God's way of family planning, would render the birth control controversy a nonissue. This natural spacing meant extra time to enjoy and focus on the present baby before the next one was born. "This would seem to be nature's way of helping us rear our little ones in an atmosphere of love and security."[9]

In addition, League members believed that breast feeding naturally enriched a father's life. They considered that most men would be both pleased and proud when their wives nursed their baby because fathers could easily realize that breast feeding was both "natural" and "womanly." Fathers, League literature emphasized, would gain confidence in realizing how much their breast-feeding wives needed their protection and support.

The League's continuing belief in the paternal benefits of breast feeding is expressed in a 1990 *New Beginnings* article about a father's confidence in the natural goodness of breast milk and his dedication to providing it for his infant. The Rookeys' family pediatrician advised ice cream to soothe their baby son's sore throat. Craig, the father, was determined that this would not mean the baby would miss out on his all-important breast milk, so he crushed a bag of his wife's frozen milk into a fine slush. Baby Christopher is reported to have loved it. The editors of the newsletter headed Craig's story with the title "All-Natural Ice Milk."[10]

The League's faith in the natural way extended to recommendations for the entire family's diet. In its earliest meetings, League leaders were concerned with extending the infant's nutritious beginning to the rest of his life. This concern, like so many other League concepts, was rooted in their trust in Providence working through Nature. "God gave man many sources of food and quality-wise, our cave-man ancestors probably had a better diet than most of us have today. Why? because they ate food in wide variety and in its natural state."[11]

More recently, La Leche League has stressed the connection between biology and behavior with a report on oxytocin. This hormone is crucial to successful breast feeding because it stimulates a mother's letdown reflex and triggers nurturing behavior. The League also claims that this hormone, which exists in higher levels in mothers who are exclusively nursing than in mothers who supplement with bottles, contributes to infant survival by "intensifying feelings of motherliness and love."[12]

THE FAMILY AS DOMESTIC CHURCH

The La Leche League ideal of family life continues to correspond to the teachings of the midcentury American Catholic Church. Among these teachings, four patterns stand out. The first two, the importance of children and a "traditionally" structured family, reflected the broad American consensus as well as American Catholic thinking. The third pattern, love as service that does not diminish the self, was and remains a more distinctively Catholic notion. Finally, the importance of Mary in the mothers' lives was the most distinctly Catholic pattern, and it is the one least acknowledged in recent League literature.

CHILDREN AT THE CENTER

From its beginning and continuing now, La Leche League has held that the domestic society, which is the nuclear family, is meant to center on children. Children, not the couple or society, are its raison d'être. In League philosophy, the needs of the mother-infant dyad take priority over all other needs and wants in the family and the community. League members are convinced that all members of the family benefit from the warmth that emanates from the relationship between a mother and her infant. Seeing the closeness of mother and baby is considered a good way to educate children for their future role as loving parents. It helps older children realize that they too came first when *they* were newborns, especially if the parents make a point of mentioning this, sharing this happy reminiscence with someone who continues to be a special part of their lives.

Very few pieces of League literature contain the assumption that a mother is bringing home a first baby, though there is a strong assumption that this may be her first breast-fed infant. Furthermore, while guiding the mother in the "art of breast feeding" is the main objective of League meetings and literature, advice about absorbing the baby into the family and meeting the continuing needs of older siblings is also an important League theme.

There is an expectation within the League that each new baby contributes to the family as a whole. Family life is enhanced, not diminished, by each new arrival. "There is a sense of joy and satisfaction on everyone's part when your newborn is settled at home, in the heart of the family. Things are as they should be — you are all together."[13] League leaders understand that liberal portions of love and reassurance go a long way toward helping an older child accept the demands of the new baby. They assure mothers that putting the needs of the baby first is actually good for older children. It helps educate them for their own future roles as parents. Leaders suggest keeping the youngest of the siblings nearby whenever the mother is nursing. In fact, among League families, establishing a "nursing corner" is a popular practice. In this space, a chair for the mom and one for the toddler are placed within reaching distance of a regularly changed assortment of play items.

The La Leche League's approach to young children differs from its approach to infants in that a toddler's or older child's wants are no longer equated with his or her needs. In the face of this stage of development, the League holds strongly to a philosophy of "loving guidance." This disciplinary approach holds that if a base of secure love was established when the child was an infant, she or he will want to act in socially approved ways. Example and sensitive suggestion will accomplish the rest. Sensitivity includes respecting the child's growth patterns while realizing that his or her inexperience requires adult direction. Parents must ease into this type of discipline from the devoted care given to infants. There is no defining moment when a sharp change occurs. Spanking and slapping are so definitely ruled out that the moral tone cannot be missed.

League material also contains narratives about the joys and struggles of caring for teenagers. League advice in these situations reflects a continuing emphasis on age-appropriate reaction and loving guidance as the focus. Narratives about raising teens tend to be idealized. Older children in League families appear to effortlessly absorb their parents' values. One League leader proudly related, "My daughter considers it the norm for babies to be near their parents at night. She also feels astonished that some mothers don't pick up their babies as soon as they cry. When she is babysitting and the mother is there, she assures them it is all right to pick up a crying baby."[14]

The League's concern for the well-being of all the children in the family is reflected in the sessions offered at its international conferences. For its twelfth conference in 1989 the League chose Anaheim, California, a location the whole family could enjoy visiting. At that conference, as at others before and since, panels covered all aspects of child development, from birth through teens. The ideas for session topics were chosen on the basis of the letters sent to the international headquarters from mothers around the world.[15] The emphasis of the importance of children to the marriage leads to a particular understanding of the roles of the spouses.

A UNIQUE UNDERSTANDING
OF COMPLEMENTARITY

In the League's earlier years, its philosophy reflected that of the culture in its expectation that fathers were breadwinners and mothers were homemakers. Such role divisions were not, however, the foundation for its concept of complementarity between spouses. League members focused on the differences in the manner in which fathers and mothers related to their children. This League focus was the opposite of what prevailed in the culture of mid-twentieth-century America. Within American society at that time, the father's public role defined his wife's. She

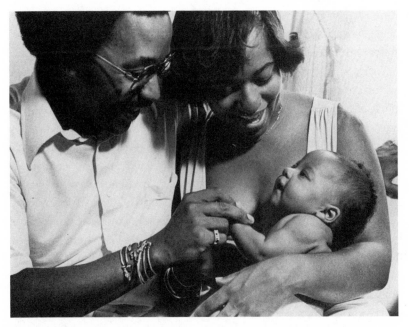

From the beginning, La Leche League members eschewed traditional role models for fathering and mothering. Both fathers and mothers are understood to have significant nurturing roles in their babies' lives.

remained within the domestic sphere in order to provide him, as well as their children, with a safe refuge. This was her contribution to his public efforts. In the La Leche community it was the mother's role that defined the father's. Because the mother-infant dyad was the center of family life and the center of community life as well, the father worked to keep it intact. Not only did he have the responsibility to be the breadwinner for his family, but he was also expected to play his own unique and active role within the family. Domestic responsibilities included helping with "chores," but they were secondary to a father's primary functions. Fathers were first expected to be "a helpmate lest the burdens of motherhood make her forget that children are a blessing; a companion because the joys of parenthood are meant to be shared." It was understood that this would call for a "reorientation" on his part "away from more self-centered pursuits of the past toward family-centered living." The founders demonstrated an awareness of the concept of "headship," but they placed a family-centered interpretation on this notion: "There is no better way to abdicate one's position as head of the family than by never being around. Just and prudent authority cannot be wielded by absentee ballot, as it were."[16]

Today, La Leche League persists in emphasizing that fathers are as important as mothers to their children but that their role is different. In 1991, *New Beginnings* carried a story that typified this perceived difference. Lon Gotsch found himself being pushed away when he reached his arms for his eight-month-old breast-fed son Kris because Kris preferred the familiar comfort of his mother's arms. Gotsch did not let this behavior daunt him. Instead, he turned Kris's shoves into a comedy routine. When the baby pushed at him, the father would tumble over backward in a great show of flailing arms and legs. This soon became a game between them that delighted Kris. More games, such as "run away from Mommy," ensued. It was not long before their games were challenging him as Kris became quicker and smarter. The Gotsches believe that their story answers the question "What are daddies for?" Fathers, according to the Gotsches, increase a child's self-esteem by giving "a child another way to see himself, reflected in Daddy's eyes."[17]

When in the 1980s more and more mothers found themselves back in the workplace, whether by necessity or choice, La Leche League philosophy expanded to accommodate the needs of these women's families; however, League members continued to understand the roles of fathers and mothers as complementary. The centrality of the mother-infant dyad did not change. The League sought creative ways to keep the employed mother and her infant together as much as possible. To accomplish this goal, League mothers turned to their husbands for help. When finances were a problem, League members objected to the father taking an additional part-time job because families require a father's presence as much as possible. Thus, assuring mother-baby togetherness often meant that both parents rearranged their work schedules so that both could share in child care.

This approach endures today. In *Sequencing*, Arlene Cardozo points out the importance of husbands being involved in their wives' choices about balancing a career with a baby. Her approach, however, remains committed to the principle of complementarity. The decision is primarily the mother's because her relationship to the baby is the focus. A father's relationship with his child is certainly at stake, but at this juncture his role is primarily one of moral and financial support. Fathers, but not mothers, are expected to be open to a spouse's decision to discontinue working outside the home while their children are young.[18]

This holding on to the complementarity principle in all circumstances drives some feminists to despair. For them, designating women as mainly responsible for child care raises unnecessary barriers to women's emancipation. The idea that child care is a mother's destiny is one Westerners are acculturated to accept. Ironically, we call it "traditional" when it is not that at all. In many more traditional cultures fathers, as well as men and women who may not even be a child's parents, care for children as successfully as mothers. Even Gabrielle Palmer, whose *Politics of Breastfeeding* is highly recommended by La Leche League, focuses on the right of employed mothers to breast-feed. She points out that in most traditional societies, the baby accompanies the mother as she works. Thus, the nursing dyad is never out of the mainstream. Breast feeding is simply something the mother of an infant does while she fulfills her major roles in society, whatever they may be. On the other hand, it can be dangerous to look to such cultures for models for our own, for whatever their child-care practices, separation of the roles of men and women tends to be fairly rigid in such societies.

FAMILY: A SAFE REFUGE FILLED WITH LOVE

In modern American culture, women need enormous support to breast-feed. Other women are not their only resource for such support. From the beginning, the founders have affirmed that an appreciative husband is a nursing mother's most powerful asset. La Leche League teaches fathers that energy and time devoted to their families provide great rewards. League father Dave Stewart wrote, "Parenting is the finest of arts, and its refinement requires a lot of conscious, unselfish effort." Stewart believed that good parenting not only makes for happy children, but that it also makes for fulfilled parents. "Ever uncertain, ever unreliable, ever unpredictable — most of life's offerings are fickle. Fatherhood is forever."[19]

League tenets, like Catholic precepts, teach that having a family will intensify the love between husband and wife. League parents Linda and Elliot Mayer testified that the birth of their daughter, Jennie, expanded their relationship. When Linda had a cesarean section, Elliot overcame the hospital nurses' objections to immediate nursing and Linda's own

fear that she did not have enough milk. As Jennie grew older, Elliot encouraged Linda's mothering strengths at those times when she saw only
her weaknesses.[20] Anne Bobman reported that one of the most romantic
times she ever experienced was a horse-and-carriage ride through the
Pennsylvania countryside that she and her husband shared with their
nursing daughter.[21]

The 1956 edition of the League manual rhapsodizes, "The miracle of
mother love is that it increases with each new birth. It is not diminished,
not limited. It is not a pie that must be sliced into smaller pieces to
accommodate extra plates at the table. With the new baby comes a re-
surgence of love for all of the family."[22]

La Leche League seeks to teach families how to provide all family
members with a safe refuge filled with love and acceptance. It does not
hold that the family can be anyone's whole life but rather that it is the
center of the rest of life. The founders acknowledged that both husband
and wife need and profit from outside interests, but they encouraged
spouses to realize that their first accountability is to their family. These
women recognized that as spouses and as parents we need aloneness as
well as togetherness, but the time spent alone ought to be directed at
enriching family life and definitely should not impoverish it.

LOVE THAT DOES NOT DIMINISH THE SELF

La Leche League's rejection of love as self-sacrifice resembles the Catholic understanding of that virtue. Although it is a commonly held notion
that the choice to breast-feed is an act of motherly self-sacrifice for the
sake of the infant, La Leche League rejects this notion. The founders
insisted that the mother who chose breast feeding embraced the joys of
mothering along with its obligations. Breast feeding provides mothers
with intense feelings of completeness and satisfaction. Early League literature frequently printed testimonies from mothers witnessing to this
principle. One mother wrote that after bottle feeding three babies, she
was struck by the immense feeling of satisfaction that her first breast-fed
baby gave her. "I feel as though I have finally arrived at motherhood."
Another mother was amazed at what a different feeling it was to be
nursing her fifth child, the first to be breast-fed. "I had no idea what I was
missing." A third mother stated that, because with her bottle-fed babies
she was free to leave whenever she wanted, she was afraid that she might

feel tied down by her breast-fed baby. In fact, she discovered that needing to be present for her infant was renewing and refreshing instead of
constricting.[23]

Donna Bryant, a former marketing manager for a large company,
related that her close friends thought that her last-minute decision to
remain at home with her first baby and not return to the job she loved
might be the result of "a hormonal imbalance." She listened to them and
returned to work, but she gradually found herself "fatigued mind, body,
and spirit." When she became pregnant with her second child, she left
work ten weeks before her due date. Friends warned that she would be
bored and would feel unproductive, but she found watching her son
grow and being there when he needed her to be the "most rewarding
work I have ever known."[24] With no intent to do so, all the mothers
quoted here align themselves against the notion that the essence of love
is self-sacrifice. For League families, love is not a duty commanded by
their roles as parents. Love of others is also love of self because loving
rewards the lover with countless benefits.

THE AGELESS APPEAL OF
MADONNA AND CHILD

For the League's founders, Mary, the mother of Jesus, exemplified such
love. The connection between La Leche League and the Catholic devotion to Mary is subtle but certainly not hidden. It radiated through the
first and second editions of *The Womanly Art of Breastfeeding*: "The security of your arms, the soft warmth of your breast, the ready comfort of
your milk, the quieting pulse of your body — all precious food to fill out
his body, quicken his soul. You are so at peace. Is not this the ageless
beauty of Madonna and Child, a time full of grace?"[25]

The organization's name originated in a title for Mary, *Nuestra Señora
de la Leche y Buen Parto* (Our Nursing Mother of Happy Delivery).
Although the religious origins of the organization's name were never
stressed, they are noted in all editions of the manual and in the official
history of the League, *The LLLove Story*. This honoring of Mary is important because in Catholic thought and popular religion through the mid-
twentieth century, Mary functioned as a model for mothers, including
the founders in their younger years. This model influenced their understanding of what it means to be a "good mother."

Child and Family, a journal edited by Herbert Ratner, was a major resource for the founders as they developed their model of good mothering. The nursing Madonna as the prototype for the "good mother" was a central theme of the *Child and Family* reprint booklet, *The Nursing Mother: Historical Insights from Art and Theology*. In this booklet, Helenka Varencov's article "The Nursing Madonna: A Cultural Motif" claims that the "Mary of the Scriptures" nursed her infant. Varencov urges Catholic mothers to imitate the nursing Madonna as an expression of devotion to her.[26] The booklet also quotes the nineteenth-century divine, Jeremy Taylor, who extolled the example of Mary. Taylor wrote, "[Mary] gave to the holy Jesus drink from those bottles which He Himself had filled for His own drinking; and her paps were as surely blessed for giving Him suck as her womb for bearing Him."[27]

La Leche League's founders express a variety of feelings and beliefs about Mary. They all remember their own mothers as being devoted to Mary, and some of them emulated their mother's devotion. Others did not. In addition, some recall having been more devoted to Mary when they were younger.

Viola Lennon never felt comfortable with devotion to Mary. She found the Rosary a confusing prayer, and Mary was not a person she could feel close to, whereas Betty Wagner never thought of herself as "a fervent person." Devotion to the Blessed Virgin, however, was the strongest Catholic influence in her life. In fact, Wagner chose to name a child after Mary because she "was an all-giving person."

Mary Ann Cahill sees Mary as "an intercessor to Christ for us. It is the mother, I think, who influences so much in the world." According to Cahill, honoring Mary, God's mother, honors God. The founders of La Leche League, she hypothesizes, were attracted to this image of the mother as honored. She herself felt drawn to the League because it reaffirmed this image. Cahill believes that it was providential that the seven founders with all their particular talents were in one place at one time, and she trusts that Our Lady of La Leche is watching over the organization and hopes it still always merits her protection. Mary Ann Kerwin remembers praying to Mary for guidance in her childhood and as a young mother. Now a lawyer, Kerwin says of Our Lady of La Leche, "It's great to have the mother of God as an advocate."

Edwina Froehlich remembers that when the founders chose the organization's name, "we kind of said, well, our Lady is certainly watching out for us and she must have inspired us." Froehlich felt any time the founders had a problem they could turn to Mary. She recalls telling herself in such situations, "Our Lady is going to help us with this." These were convictions that she had held from childhood. As a young girl, Edwina had learned that Mary "always had God's ear." She and the other founders believed that Mary "understood about women. It was just kind of a sort of natural thing for us when we were dealing with female things to think in terms of the mother of God."

Mary White has had "a lifelong devotion to Mary as the mother of Jesus." She believes that Mary "must have something we are expected to look up to." White holds that Mary had, as all mothers do, special challenges. Yet, in the face of these challenges, Mary remained "close to her Son, patient, loving, and gentle." White is "glad we have Our Lady as a model" because Mary was humble despite her chosen role as God's mother.

Marian Tompson emphasizes this aspect of Mary's image. Mary was a model, "someone to imitate," precisely because she had experienced "all the troubling times" that all mothers do. Tompson envisions Mary as "a real person with real needs." Because Mary appeared to her this way, Tompson always felt Mary was "someone to turn to" in her own struggles.[28]

SHINING A LIGHT IN THE DARKNESS

La Leche League began with a social outreach agenda. In the manner of Catholic action groups, League groups worked to transform the world. This approach endures. Today's members take seriously their responsibility to see that there is a League "for the next generation of mothers, babies, and families."[29] These women see themselves as part of an organization that has changed attitudes not just toward breast feeding but toward all of family life.[30] As leader Patti White states, "The circle of love has been an ever-broadening one for me." White credits the League with preparing her and her husband not only to love their children but also to care for all the needy persons who came into their lives.[31]

The concepts that guide La Leche League's approach to family life reflect two aspects of the Catholic perception that the family functions as a "light to the world." League families strive both to be models of "good" family life and actively to promote better family life in the community at large. These two aspects are understood as intertwined modes of action within the work of the association.

Soon after the organization began, Herbert Ratner declared, "Deep down in your hearts you know that if you do a good job on the women who are interested in breastfeeding, their fine example will change the world." Ratner compared the women of La Leche League to an order of nuns who worked serving the poor. Those women, he held, served the poor because they felt Christ's call in their hearts, not because of a rationalized ideology. The religious sisters were, Ratner believed, as unconcerned with political arguments over the relative merits of capitalism and communism as they were uninterested in Leo XIII's encyclical on social justice. He told the women of La Leche League that, like these nuns, they served those who needed help desperately because they perceived "the need and could not turn away." Ratner assured them, "Your work is really a kind of corporal work of mercy."[32]

For Viola Lennon, Catholicism was "all about how Christianity was coming into the world and lifting up creation," and her involvement in the Christian Family Movement was the training ground for her work in the League. Mary Ann Cahill recalled, "We did pattern the League quite a bit after CFM. When you think of CFM, you met in home; you had, what, a leader. When one group was getting rather large, you broke off with another." At the time of La Leche League's beginnings, there were several active CFM groups in Franklin Park. Mary and Greg White were the leaders of the group to which several League founders belonged, including Marian Tompson, who would become the League's first president. Tompson "enjoyed the theology of action, the energy of the group, and the belief that you can make a difference," which the CFM brought to her family. The CFM encouraged her to see needs and do something about them. This was the League approach from the beginning. The founders assumed that, if they helped families, their actions would help the community and thus the world. Tompson recalls thinking, "So, it's worth taking the time despite our misgivings."

Froehlich also discerns certain CFM influences on the League. For one thing, they shared the same model of intervention. When the first nucleus of the founders came together, Froehlich recalls, "We had already *observed* that these women needed help. It was all from the beginning, *action*." The *judgment*, she believes, was the founders' understanding that they had both breast-feeding knowledge and the ability to share it, "so let's let it be known we're here." Also, the CFM taught Froehlich to trust in Providence. "If this is what God wants us to do, it's going to go and we'll just do it. Whatever we know how to do, we'll do. And if this is part of God's plan, then it'll work. And if it doesn't, then either it's not His plan or we're not the right ones to do it and He'll give it to somebody else."

On a different note, Tompson stresses that, whereas the first stirrings of the ideas for the League began at a CFM picnic, it "is not whose picnic it was" that was important. What counted was the illumination that came out of it, that women labored under the unfairness "of the loss of their right to breast-feed."[33]

The example that League families established at that picnic is central to the La Leche League tradition. Continuing down to the present day, leaders and members the world over continue to endeavor to establish a pattern for the "good" family. One founding mother saw herself and her fellow founders as apostles and the group mothers as disciples who, in turn, go out and "teach all nations."[34]

La Leche League members hope to see breast feeding become the cultural norm. They believe that example is their best tool. Because society was not yet supportive of nursing mothers, in a 1988 article for *New Beginnings* Gwen Gotsch, senior editor for LLLI Publications, urged League members to demonstrate how easily and discreetly a baby can be nursed in public. Some may claim, she realized, that such behavior is fanatical. In fact, the surgeon general's report of 1983 made breast feeding a national health priority. Gotsch insisted that the mother who breast-fed in public contributed to this national endeavor by making nursing an open practice. She entreated nursing mothers to take their baby along and nurse in every type of public place from churches to amusement parks. Their example, she believed, "will show others that you can enjoy and nurture your baby through breastfeeding and still lead an active life. So go ahead, be a fanatic. No one ever said that changing an entire culture was going to be easy."[35]

In a 1989 article, Costa Rican Betty Lewis also discussed changing attitudes about where the mother-child dyad belonged. Because managerial accounting, a class Lewis needed, was being offered when her breast-fed daughter was only one month old, she was able to obtain permission to bring her daughter, Carolina, to class. At first, Lewis left class whenever the baby cried, but soon other students protested. Some even held the baby for her to give her a break. Lewis learned from this experience that, if mothers are determined to nurse their babies, they should not let themselves be restricted by fear of what others might think. "No matter where we live, we must take charge of our lives and decide for ourselves what is important."[36]

Living by League principles, members hold, changes more than just infant nurturing practices. Leader Patti White and her husband, the parents of three children, have worked in rehabilitation programs in Amsterdam and with the street children of São Paulo, Brazil. In a 1991 article, Patti stated that being a League member gave her the experience she needed in her work. Also, nearly every person who lived in the centers where the Whites worked told them that they had learned how to be a family from watching the Whites relate to each other.[37]

League fathers are major contributors to the organization's efforts to change the world. When Mark Everman was awarded special recognition by his company for his work, he received a trip for two to accompany other rewarded employees to a resort for four days. When he asked about bringing his toddler son, Kevin, he was told it would be "inappropriate." Despite pressure to attend so as to demonstrate his "team spirit," Everman declined the trip. In the end, the company, impressed by his dedication, gave the family three round-trip airfares in place of the vacation. The Evermans hoped the incident would influence the management to take into account the needs of their employees' families when they gave out future awards.[38]

SECULAR MISSION, RELIGIOUS IMPULSE

Despite the resemblance between the beliefs and practices of American Catholicism and those of La Leche League, the League is not now, nor has it ever been, officially or even casually affiliated with the Catholic Church. This reality is due to a conscious decision on the part of the founders. Yet the impulse behind the decision reflects Christian action at its best. Wishing to help any mother who needed them, the founders emphasized their secular mission so that no one would feel excluded. None of the founders recalls making this decision formally. There was simply a feeling from the beginning, Froehlich recalls, that "we didn't want to be a religious group."

Mary White, however, comprehends the League's beginnings as having "a somewhat religious overtone." She recognizes that understanding nature as a guide to "being on the right road" has roots in Catholic thought. The Catholicism of the founders, she believes, functioned as "a reminder of things we thought were important." She also holds that the fact that the League needs to appeal to a wide range of families "should not mean that we cannot mention our faith." Over time, however, the League has moved away from any religious language. The impetus, White states, came from the publication department, which "is always very nervous about religious overtones." One of the early November–December issues had so many stories focused on Christmas that the editor at the time, Mary Carson, insisted that a no-religious-language policy be made official. White has never felt completely comfortable with this decision. "They practically had us denying the existence of God." She declares, "I hope we are not a Godless organization!"

Froehlich reports that in the beginning some of the mothers who came to the meeting asked questions about church teachings. "For example, we went through the era when the Catholic Church was advocating large families. And people would write to us and say, 'I understand all of you people have large families.'" Froehlich believes these mothers worried that if having large families was integral to League membership, they would not be able to belong. To dispel these misconceptions, the founders stressed that even though most of their families were large, "having a large family is up to you. Whether you want one or ten children, we are here to help you."

Froehlich recalls that some community members even told new mothers not to attend League meetings because it was a group "run by the Pope," whose members were strict Catholics interested in propagating their faith through the organization. Other factors contributed to the perception of the League as a Catholic organization. Although Froehlich is convinced that the Catholicism of the founders was a coincidence of friendship and family ties, the early meetings attracted Catholics because the Catholic community of that time was close-knit. The earliest article about La Leche League appeared in a Catholic family magazine. As Froehlich points out, since the magazine's circulation was limited because it was Catholic, there was a strong Catholic response to the article. Altogether, these factors began to bring home the need to stress the League's non-Catholic goals and to focus on the central issue, good mothering through breast feeding.

Viola Lennon stresses that, although La Leche League is far from a "Godless organization," from the beginning some attending mothers came from non-Catholic faith communities, so shortly after its inception, League membership was no longer predominantly Catholic. Because many of the women seeking help came from different faiths, Lennon believes "our path was almost dictated from the beginning." The fact that women from many different backgrounds sought help from the League led to an early decision to avoid the use of religious language in League materials. As soon as the founders established an advisory board that included other leaders, they purposely sought women with Protestant and Jewish backgrounds. Despite the many faiths represented on the board, the name for the organization remained without objections about its religious origin.

Because the decision to be a secular organization was made so early, when leaders explained the origin of the name, they emphasized that the name had been chosen to avoid offending the sensibilities of the time. This emphasis was needed, Betty Wagner maintains, because all the founders were Catholic. As a group of Catholic people who had given their organization one of Mary's titles, they very quickly had to demonstrate that the organization had nothing to do with religion, that its focus was breast feeding. Wagner recognizes that for some time at the beginning, the religious origins of the founders did color how people looked at the League because people in Franklin Park, which was a small town at the time, knew they were Catholic. As the League stressed over and over their basic message of good mothering through breast feeding, mothers were able to see that the League accepted everyone.

Mary Ann Kerwin maintains that although the founders never saw the League as a Catholic group, they lived in such a Catholic environment that it affected who would originally come to meetings. By the time they had incorporated as a not-for-profit and nonsectarian organization, however, they had already been questioned about their Catholicism and had made clear that they were not a Catholic group. It was essential to the founders to put across this notion because "we wanted to help *all mothers* who wished to breast-feed." This stated, Kerwin believes that it is a mistake to leave all religious language and all reference to the founders' Catholicism out of League publications. For Kerwin, this amounts to "rewriting history." Since the choice to drop any religious language was made "after the network was in place," Kerwin worries that it alienates the

League from its origins. Many mothers have told Kerwin that they "feel a deep spirituality in their connection and involvement with La Leche League." She does not believe this is mere coincidence.

ABORTION: A LONG, AGONIZING, DIFFICULT ARGUMENT

One central Catholic concern, abortion, has caused dissent within the leadership of La Leche League. Some of the members believed that the League should take a prolife stance. They saw this as consistent with the fact that the League has not confined its discussion to breast feeding but has branched out into other areas of infant welfare. As Mary White has said, "If we want what is best for children from conception on, we should say we are for life." Although White received a standing ovation when she included this position in her keynote address to a La Leche League conference in the late 1970s, the advisory board called for her resignation.

Froehlich recalls that, for the board, abortion was the subject of "many a long, agonizing, difficult argument and discussion." One of the problems raised was that many of the accredited leaders were in favor of choice. These women had joined the League with the understanding that being prolife was not required of them. Also, as Froehlich notes, the League did not appeal to "an elite little group of Catholic women. We were dealing with mothers all over." Some mothers did write to ask that the League support the prolife movement, and, Froehlich recalls, Ratner wanted the League to attend·to their pleas. It was the only time, she relates, that any of the founders were in conflict with Ratner. These women believed that the abortion issue was too complex to be settled in a few statements and that the League was not "equipped to deal" with it. They did not wish to detract from the League's central message. This position became the prevailing one, and the organization has no official stance on abortion. It is an issue leaders are counseled to avoid.[39]

While this very volatile issue is avoided, all the League's other convictions about family life remain firmly embedded in its contemporary praxis. League members understand breast feeding to be the natural means to a good beginning in parenting. Good parenting includes not only the care of children but also a constant replenishing of spousal love. Within such families, the League believes, both family members and others can find haven from an uncaring world, but such havens are not understood as escapes. League members believe that the world can be transformed and that they have both the obligation and the ability to effect such a transformation. The roots of these convictions lie within Catholic understandings of family life. In League praxis, these convictions intertwine with members' confidence that the League's principles of infant nutrition are more adequate than much medical advice offered to new mothers and with their certainty that even the most accurate scientific information cannot replace a strong woman-to-woman network for the sharing of child-care information.

chapter 8

· ·

Asking the Hard Questions

La Leche League praxis can be viewed and engaged critically from three perspectives: its active, reflective, and creative aspects.[1] This chapter addresses the balance among these various aspects of La Leche League.

INADEQUACY OF REFLECTIVE ACTIVITY

Although the League has always engaged in some reflective activity, it has focused its attention on the active and creative facets of its work. Consequently, those elements within its philosophy that receive careful scrutiny are forceful and convincing. They include the League's understanding of the science of infant nutrition, its sensitivity to the physical, psychological, and social needs of new mothers, and its discernment regarding effective group and one-on-one counseling.

Other equally active and creative elements of League theory and practice receive little critical attention and are, therefore, less commanding and more vulnerable to negative critique. These elements span all areas of the League's work with families. First, in its use of the sciences, the League tends toward an unexamined identification of certain perceived needs and tendencies of infants and their mothers as moral imperatives. Second, the League's understanding of the existential situation of contemporary women errs toward an unwarranted optimism. Third, League materials demonstrate an unreflective use of the words "nature" and "natural." Finally, League members are overly confident that spousal mutuality can exist where traditionally defined gender roles are maintained. The work of this chapter is to examine those claims in League beliefs that need more critically reflective attention.

Both the well-scrutinized and the unreflective elements of the League's theory-practice interaction are based on metaphors that attempt to describe what kind of universe we live in. These metaphors both lay the foundation for and interact with the ethical theories that underlie La Leche League's writings and its interaction with families. Despite their importance, they receive no reflective attention within League literature. It is not that the League's beliefs and approach are entirely inappropriate; instead, it is that some of its claims were developed unsystematically and without using a wide variety of disciplinary approaches. Yet, in all historical activity, the three aspects of praxis overlap and form a single thrust even though at different moments the participants may engage one aspect more than they do the other two.

ENGAGING IN A CRITICAL REFLECTION

La Leche League's unscrutinized tenets and practices call for a clarifying moment of reflection. Such scrutiny uncovers for us the metaphors that underlie the League's praxis and illuminates the strengths and the weaknesses of the moral ground of League concepts and practices. We can then see La Leche League as a community that has a history of dialogue with other communities. The dialogue has served to enhance the practical wisdom that has emerged from the life of the community. In addition, we find that integrating metaphors exist across the full spectrum of the League's work. These metaphors share a specific characteristic: all are dialectical—that is, they express the tensions, paradoxes, and ambiguities of the human situation. Finally, our exploration allows us to acknowledge the enhanced goal that inspires the League today. The goal is strong loving families that are committed to working for a better life for all families everywhere.

BREAST FEEDING:

A SACRED ACTIVITY FOR A PROFANE WORLD

Mircea Eliade declares that for the persons capable of religious experience all nature reveals itself as cosmic sacrality.[2] For the women of La Leche League, breast feeding's very identification with the natural renders it a revelation of the sacred in the midst of a profane world. Although only the League's earliest literature contains explicitly religious language, the deep metaphors that have grounded its philosophy from the beginning remain implicit. Such metaphors permeate all of the League's practices and beliefs, which we have explored in the preceding chapters.

PROMPTINGS OF THE HEART

The League's relationship to science reveals metaphors on which the League draws to promote a particular theory of infant development and to justify a vast array of precepts about family life. In the view of Herbert Ratner, the mid-twentieth-century medical community devoted enormous resources to developing bottled infant formulas while ignoring "the fact that species-specific breast milk had had the longest clinical trial of any food ever made for the young." This ignorance, he believed, pitted physicians against nature. The League presented an alternative. Its adherents looked not to science and technology but to nature as the repository of wisdom. "They did not entrust the development of the mother-infant relationship to the vagaries of scientific advance, but rather, they placed their faith in nature and the promptings of the heart, a mode by which nature communicates many teachings."[3]

In the twenty-five years between the publication of the first and the third editions of the League's manual, there occurred a dramatic return to breast feeding for which the League takes at least partial credit. As Ratner and the League perceived it, during this period medical science used dramatic new findings to contribute positively to the establishment and acceptance of breast feeding. The League willingly used such information to promote its cause. In Ratner's opinion, however, an opinion that carried great weight in the association, "What nursing mothers did by natural inclination and intuition, and learned experientially, scientists corroborated experimentally."[4]

Thus, even as the League acquired masses of specific and well-docu-mented scientific evidence, this was never viewed as anything but a ver-ification of what League mothers had believed all along. Their first act of faith was taking the position that breast feeding is in itself good. The League understands meeting an infant's needs as the basis for all further physical and psychological health. League teachings reflect a confidence that basic human biological tendencies provide us with empirically dis-cernible truth claims. Only secondarily do members place their trust in science to confirm this faith.

In addition to limiting their acceptance of scientific findings to those findings that cohered with already well-defined principles, League women focused their faith on an approach to infant care that stemmed from these findings and principles. This school of thought insisted that breast milk is so far superior to infant formula that only the most extreme conditions call for the introduction of any formula into a baby's diet.

This position also stressed that the infant's psychological well-being depended on the almost constant proximity of his or her mother for several months after birth. The League understands these as scientific concepts that justify a particular mothering approach.

Critical reflection on this justification raises two areas of concern. First, although many child development specialists regard healthy pre-oedipal experiences as optimum for the development of a firm and cohe-sive self-identity, it is also widely recognized that other factors beyond this period may be equally influential. These include the multitude of experiences associated with living in a highly differentiated and mobile society. Thus, even if the ideal mother-child rapport could be achieved, factors beyond the mother's control may play havoc with the security and trust her care has instilled. In favor of the League's stance, however, research into infant development indicates that meeting an infant's needs is so basic to future growth that later attempts to provide this foundation may not be totally successful.[5]

Second, the League's confidence in this approach to child nurturance does not rely solely on science. The League's official logo is a mother cradling her infant drawn in gracefully enfolding lines that mark the mother and baby as one. Such an image easily brings to mind many other representations of transcendent femaleness. Such images have pre-historical roots but would have been most familiar to the League found-ers in the many artistic depictions of the Madonna. Since such exposure is not limited to Catholic women, nor to the past, a widespread and deeply rooted metaphor of motherhood inclined League mothers to a specific scientific approach to infant care and to mothering in general.

The broader scientific and cultural community challenges both an absolute acceptance of "breast is best" and an insistence on mother-infant proximity. New mothers continue to be counseled, as they were in the 1950s, that although breast milk is the *preferred* infant food, mothers can rest assured that whichever method they choose, their infant will thrive. Expectant mothers are warned that breast feeding will tie them to the baby because they will have to be available whenever the baby is hungry. Breast pumps are listed as essential equipment, regardless of whether the mother plans to return to work. In other words, mother-baby proximity is actually viewed by some members of the wider community as a disadvantage of breast feeding. In addition, the superiority of breast milk is questioned. Dr. Alvin Eden, chairman of the department of pediatrics at Wyckiff Heights Medical Center in Brooklyn, New York, states emphatically that formula feeding is a perfectly acceptable alternative to breast feeding.[6]

Thus, one could argue that, faced with the strong counterclaims of the surrounding culture, League members seek in scientific theory a foundation and an anchor for the moral choices they are making. In doing so, they convert some scientific theories into myth. This way of relating the "heart's reasons" to the mind's reasons has a long history in Christian thought.[7] Catholic doctrine, while upholding the good of rational thought, has resisted any interpretation of reality that gives reason precedence over faith. Shortly after the League's founding, John XXIII expressed his concern that because religious education was slighted in comparison with scientific education, science had gained an extraordinary influence on the contemporary culture to the detriment of the quality of human life.[8] Catholic understandings posit that scientific findings, like those of medical science and divine natural law grounded in human instincts and experience, give reciprocal help.

BREAST FEEDING: A UNIVERSAL RIGHT

Underlying religioethical metaphors also appear when the League communicates its convictions. La Leche League exists as a response to an anxiety specifically engendered by the modern technological culture, the

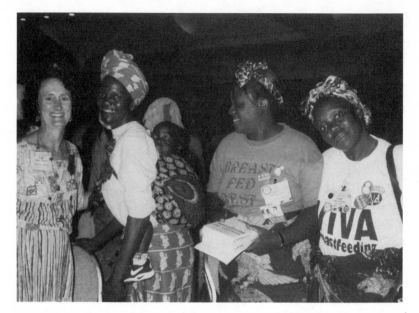

Because La Leche League has reached out to mothers worldwide, its conventions are attended by women of many nations who are joined by their determination that all children everywhere receive the best nurturing possible.

difficulty many contemporary women experience in their attempt to nurse their infants. The League believes that were it not for an intrusive culture, a woman's natural instincts would enable her to make morally correct choices about infant and child care. This ability, the League believes, is intrinsic to a woman's embodiment as female.

The League holds that this intrusive culture has interfered with the birthright of an infant to his or her own mother's milk and the mother's right to nourish her own infant. "The League views itself as the baby's advocate."[9] For the League, these rights are essential components of a just society. Thus, League principles and the actions grounded in these perceived rights carry an implicit moral determination to right a wrong. This sense of obligation is itself embedded in a claim to meaning and truth. For League members, babies' basic needs are unchanging, regardless of when or where they are born. Breast feeding seems to them to be "a small miracle, belonging rightfully to mothers, babies, and families the world over."[10] The quasi-religious roots of this claim are, however, never made explicit in League literature. League writers focus on examining scientific claims and their impact on the League's concepts and practices. Thus, League writings generate universal moral claims for truth based on perceived scientific facts without understanding how such moral precepts have expanded into a full range of fundamental claims about the ethics of family life.

Respect for the various situations individual mothers face is central to the functioning of the local groups. The League's literature and the multiple sessions of their international conventions address the multiplicity of family, medical, and national situations in which mothers find themselves. In all of this analysis, the assumption of the baby's right to his or her mother's milk is never questioned. That circumstances may interfere is acknowledged but always with the presumption that ignorance and a lack of support by the medical community, not the mother's inability to breast-feed, are the obstacles to be overcome. The League acknowledges only certain extremely rare medical situations that may preclude breast feeding.[11]

In the past, the League has failed to face the complexity of broader contextual impediments that mothers face worldwide. More recently, the League has confronted these situations with innovative new programs. The underlying assumption, however, remains that every baby is born with the "right" to his or her mother's milk.

LA LECHE LEAGUE AND THE
NEW REALISM IN FEMINIST THOUGHT

Contemporary feminists are exploring motherhood with a new realism. They are discerning and accepting the powerful bonds and enormous responsibilities of being "also a mother." At the same time, calling for new families that reflect the present needs of both parents and their children, they are seeking an alternative to the traditional approach to parenting. They ask that the nonparenting public understand that society as a whole benefits when all citizens share to some degree the responsibilities involved in raising healthy, successful children. Many feminists no longer fear being advocates for children and for families. Instead, they have developed several strategies for coping with their two-career lives. Not all of these strategies are successful. Many need continuing refinement. Feminists see a real need to engage nonparents in their struggle and work toward that aim.

Recently, La Leche League has also developed a broader approach to questions of mothering in contemporary times. The League has always held that there is no essential conflict between the needs of women and those of their children. In addition, it believes that mother-baby closeness need not interfere with women's accomplishments in the public sphere. Like feminists, League members comprehend that societal structures can serve as wedges between a woman and her infant or young child. Unlike many contemporary feminists, however, they are more likely to insist on solutions that minimize the separation of mothers and infants. They focus on solutions such as sequencing the at-home and professional phases of their life cycle, working at home, and taking children to the workplace. Nevertheless, there exists in the League's ideology a tendency to overestimate women's ability to overcome the biases against the "mommy track." The League also underestimates the actual economic desperation of many employed mothers. Although the League publication *The Heart Has Its Own Reasons* contains many inspiring stories of families that have endured straightened circumstances in order to allow the mother to remain with the children, these were stories of families with two parents in which the father was employed. Thus, a continuing difference in perceptions keeps feminists and League members in different arenas, both advocating a better family life but taking different, and often conflicting, positions.

MARY AND LA LECHE LEAGUE:
A COMPLEX RELATIONSHIP

At the subconscious center of this conflict between La Leche League praxis and that of contemporary feminism stands a symbol of motherhood, the Madonna as the traditional mother in Western thought. For the founders of the League, the Madonna, familiar since childhood, was most powerfully represented by Nuestra Señora de la Leche y Buen Parto. Consequently, this image also serves as a metaphor for mothering within the League. The power of this image must be envisioned in order to understand both the League's perception of what it means to be a woman and the feminist critique of this perception.

Devotion to Mary is one of the most popular and original characteristics of Catholic Christianity. Mary's place in Catholicism has a multitude of interpretations, but the fact of the massive devotion to Mary cannot be denied. In the years since the founding of La Leche League, however, the image of Mary has undergone a major transition. Only fourteen years after the dogma of the Assumption was defined, Vatican II encouraged the leaders of the Catholic Church to take "as far as it was feasible . . . the 'minimalist' line in Marian thinking."[12]

Like the official Catholic hierarchy, some League founders now minimize the part Marian devotions play in their lives and its influence on League thinking. Originally, the founders did make a devotional choice in naming La Leche League. They "thought the group would stay small; we looked for Our Lady's protection and we liked our link to her."[13] Later, the unexpected growth of the League and its appeal to women from diverse religious backgrounds caused the founders and other early leaders to disregard Mary's significance to their group.

An exploration of the symbol of Mary as revealed in Scripture and Catholic tradition, though, opens up the possibility that this symbol remains a powerful influence on the League. Michael Whelan, president of the Catholic Theological Union, in Sydney, Australia, examined the many ways the symbol of Mary works as an expression of the covenant between God and the people of God. Four of these correspond with La Leche League's vision of life within its community. These correspondences offer insight into the strengths of this image. First, Mary joyfully participates in Catholics' pilgrimage of faith. She set an example of one who questions, challenges, pursues, and searches. As Catholic Christians, the founding mothers are seekers who question and challenge while holding fast to a fixed set of core beliefs. Second, Mary suffered as only a mother can. Having given everything she was to her child, she stood by Jesus as he chose his own tragic path. Mary is the model of the mother who meets the child's needs on the child's terms. League mothers, in conflict with much "expert" advice, care for their children in rhythm with the children's perceived needs, often sacrificing their own tendencies to this cause.

Third, Mary's presence at Pentecost was the ultimate expression of motherly "thereness." Just as she bore into existence the enfleshed Word of God, so she parents and loves the community of God.[14] For Catholics, Mary "represents the human insight that the Ultimate is passionately tender, seductively attractive, irresistibly inspiring, and graciously healing."[15] In this same tradition, the women of La Leche League center their work on nurturing family life by helping mothers to nurture their own families. La Leche League wisdom contains a deep interest in the well-being of all humankind, which League members believe is a manifestation of women's motherly wisdom.

Fourth, for Whelan, Mary is a paradox. She loves without possessing, remains faithful but continues to question, accepts and challenges her children, is always there but does not intrude, supports without intruding, is self-denying yet self-possessed, and knows how to be both gentle and determined.[16] League mothers love fully, but their final goal is their child's independence. They hold firmly to League ideals but remain open to the opinions of parents and professionals. They stay by new mothers but seek to help them find their own answers. League mothers are willing to sacrifice much for the sake of their families, yet they are very proud of all their public accomplishments. League mothers seldom raise their voices, but it is impossible to turn them away from their mission to render breast feeding a universal mothering experience.

These are the positive aspects of Mary's symbolic image, but this image also has its weaknesses. Because La Leche League has chosen to push the Marian image to the margins of its awareness, the negative interpretations implicit in this model invisibly intertwine themselves into League concepts. These are the very aspects of Mary as symbol that are most vulnerable to feminist critique. Often they are also the facets of League practice and belief that present the greatest contrast to feminist thought.

The most frequent critique of the Marian symbol has been its perceived passivity. As Kari Borresen has noted, in classical Christology the "father's role—filled in the case of Christ by the Holy Spirit—was seen as active, while the mother's role was passive."[17] Generations of Catholics have seen in Mary's femininity a humility and receptivity that binds women to a passive role in the community, in the church, and in the family.[18] The church has continually portrayed Mary as passive and submissive, a portrayal that contrasts with the scriptural narrative, where Mary appeared as a strong, courageous woman.[19]

A second weakness in the Marian image is that Mary "is always presented to us as a relational or 'hyphen' being, in other words, as someone who is always closely connected with someone else."[20] Within the League, women are valued for their individual contributions but are always seen within the context of their family or their League group. All the founders of La Leche League are both strong women and unique individuals. Yet the biographies of these women included in the second and third editions of the manual gave names of husbands and of children. These biographies related the multiple functions that each woman had performed within the League, but what the women did before they became mothers was not mentioned, nor did readers learn what other interests they might have outside the League and their families.

LA LECHE LEAGUE'S UNDERSTANDING
OF THE NATURE OF WOMEN

There is a central paradox to good mothering through breast feeding. It is a biological function of the female body that most mammals in most situations perform successfully by instinct. Yet, at the same time, like pregnancy and childbirth, in certain circumstances it becomes wrought with complications that threaten its success.

This paradox often places La Leche League in a quandary. The women of the League fully acknowledge that breast feeding is a learned art. Despite this recognition, they also wish to claim for mothers a certain instinctual knowledge, something that gives them an edge over expert advice, something particularly womanly. The second edition of the manual warns, "Read as much as you like, but always remember to rely *most* on your own motherly instincts, taking into account your own and your family's particular personality differences, likes and dislikes, and so on. Don't try to do every[thing] 'by the book.' Just relax and be a mother."[21] This approach can be appreciated as morally responsible. It asks mothers to be aware of their own agency and their capacity to contemplate more than one course of action.[22] On the other hand, this approach includes an implicit trust that mothers know some things by virtue of being mothers, that is, by their very nature.

Feminist theologians have observed several problems with such trust. First, perceptions about motherhood result largely from the socialization process. These authors claim that motherliness is not natural to women but is learned like any other social skill. As young girls, female children until very recently were expected to play with toys that geared them toward a domestic role. As today's women grew older they were encouraged to focus on making themselves attractive so that they might attract a man. The highest dream of adolescence was to become a wife and mother, and although today's adolescent girls are expected to prepare to earn an income, attracting males is still a central focus of much adolescent literature. As a result of this socializing process, young women enter the marital partnership expecting to be primarily responsible for making their marriage work and their home a happy one. Thus, the adult woman is so completely socialized to her expected role that it actually "feels" natural. These expectations have been so universalized in Western culture that an individual woman's convictions are bolstered by those of her surrounding community. It may seem that certain aspects of a woman's parenting role, such as pregnancy, childbirth, and lactation, are determined solely by biology. The meanings these aspects carry in a given society, however, are culturally determined. Significantly, such cultural determination includes the extent to which these segments of a woman's life limit both her domestic power and her participation in the public arena. The central question is, should biological roles direct the full scope of a woman's life?

Second, feminist theologians have noted that the assumption of a single women's nature sees all women as different from men and the same as each other. In reality, however, women's differences from one another are as significant as their differences from men. Gender cannot be analyzed on its own. It is also true that each woman's mothering experience, while it encompasses some form of mother-child relationship, is separable from the kind of woman she is. Only the imperatives of infant needs remain despite maternal differences. The challenge is to determine how a mother can maximize the needs of her child without making them the exclusive arbitrator of her own fulfillment as a person. A third problem is noted by Christine Gudorf, who observed that similarly close attention is rarely given to "the nature of men, of fatherhood, and of masculinity."[23] Such neglect was not a part of League ideology. Within the League, concentrated attention is given to questions of fatherhood and masculinity, although League perceptions of both motherhood and fatherhood were understood as rooted in nature rather than in culture.

Feminist theologians have also criticized the tendency of the Catholic Church to understand women who seek to expand their horizons beyond the family as being selfish and uncaring. This is a serious challenge. The League must be careful to deflect accusations that it supports such perceptions. In their concern for supporting the family, several popes accused women of abandoning their natural selflessness for selfishness. In addition, church leaders expressed the fear that feminism would demolish women's redemptive capacity for suffering.[24] La Leche League has never claimed suffering as a virtue in women. In practice, the very threat of an unconscious acceptance of such concepts jeopardizes the League's claim that women have unique functions to fulfill in family and in community life. The League needs to reflect critically on such claims if it is to overcome the skepticism that many feminists direct at any avowal that women are essentially different from men and that all women share this uniqueness.

Susan Okin argued in *Justice, Gender, and the Family* that typical American family life was not "conducive to the rearing of citizens with a strong sense of justice." Okin held that, when women construct their lives around being the primary parent, they become vulnerable to the unjust socioeconomic consequences of gender-structured marriages. Allowing the inner workings of family life to be something that people are left to work out for themselves can lead to injustice. Because choices within families have repercussions, just principles need to be developed to govern these choices. The question of women's roles in the family and in society "belongs both to the sphere of 'the good' and to that of 'the right.'" For justice to prevail, men and women need to share equally in all paid and unpaid work and in productive and reproductive labor. To achieve this goal, we can make no assumptions about what is a man's or a woman's role. For men and women to be equally responsible for domestic life and child care, childbearing must be conceptually separated from child rearing. How much time a child spends with a given parent must be determined without reference to the parent's maleness or femaleness.[25]

Feminists such as Okin present a grave challenge to La Leche League. Clearly, for a woman who is breast-feeding her infant and who understands this not just as a feeding technique but as a way of mothering, child rearing cannot be conceptually separated from childbearing or from lactation. Okin was correct to claim that new theories of justice that do not consider gender are totally unsatisfactory. La Leche League, however, also raises several questions about justice in the family. It asks, for instance, why society does not value parental nurture as "meaningful work." League mothers also challenge the equating of "parental equality" with "equal" time. Another important question the League raises is, "Does a difference in parental roles necessarily imply family injustice?" Is there not also an imbalance if a parent gives and withholds certain parenting behavior according to an abstract concept of justice rather than according to the valid needs of both parent and child?

These are valid questions. Yet, at the same time, La Leche League cannot ignore feminist concerns. It is possible that League mothers could broaden their praxis so as to acknowledge feminist anxieties without compromising their own principles. For instance, they could free their image of motherhood from naively essentialist claims about its nature. There are other, more penetrating claims they could make. The League's image of motherhood offers many women very real possibilities for a creative, caring, and fulfilling mothering experience. Also, the League disputes the contention that remaining at home with her infant and very young children limits a woman's full expression of self. It argues that it is society's image of the at-home mother that needs to be altered. Struggling to effect such perceptual changes would be difficult, but the League's strength lies in its child-focused approach. League members are fully aware that an infant's developmental needs are not as adaptable as a society's rules and roles. Later therapeutic attempts to achieve developmental steps missed in infancy can be difficult, if not impossible. Third, the League could benefit from a better understanding of the way gender is reproduced from one generation to the next. The real experiences of women must be included in the dialogue between the League and feminism. As women, League members need to move beyond a fear of difference. Doing so requires giving up attempts to conceptually universalize the situation of women vis-à-vis Western cultural assumptions. At the same time, the very real satisfaction so many women have found in parenting the La Leche League way cannot be ignored.

LA LECHE LEAGUE AND A
RELIGIOUS ETHIC OF FAMILY LIFE

Logically speaking, a system of practical moral reasoning can develop independently of religion. Yet, in its full embodiment, a set of moral precepts — like La Leche League's ten basic concepts — is grounded in metaphors given sacred valence by those who live by its rules. La Leche League employs vast personal experience and abundant scientific research to ground its theories of obligation. It utilizes effectively a multinational woman-to-woman network to communicate its convictions. It does not, however, recognize the quasi-religious undercurrents of these sources of information and power. Because religious language has been a controversial issue for League leaders, the League overlooks the religiously grounded ethic of family life that empowers its members and enables them to adhere to practices and beliefs that often contradict contemporary culture's view of family life. Lack of acknowledgment leads to lack of critical reflection. Thus, League principles and actions are vulnerable to both misinterpretation and stagnation. A fresh look at natural law theory and neighbor love reveals a more authentic and more open understanding of the League's family ethic.

JUST WHAT IS "NATURAL" MOTHERING?

La Leche League materials make rather sweeping and uncritical use of the words "nature" and "natural" to justify the kind of mothering they support. As used in League literature, these terms are variously shaded toward a scientific tone, reflect a romantic notion of a benevolent Nature, or make the claim, as did the first edition of the manual, that breast feeding is "God's way of doing things." La Leche League's intermixing of divergent metaphorical applications of "nature" and "natural" reproduces the perplexities apparent in religiously based ethical theories about the existence of a natural law. The popes since Leo XIII have offered a view of humanity in which two aspects of human nature are revealed. First, humans were considered as united by their common possession of reason. All humans, the pontiffs assumed, desired truth naturally, and all were aware of natural moral law. The popes also held that a benign nature reflected God's own beneficent intentions. The founders tended to place the psychobiological tendencies and needs of parents and children into a narrative and moral context that assumed this natural law and a benign Providence. In doing so, they were unconsciously caught in the uncertain ramifications of juxtaposing a traditional Catholic emphasis on a universal human nature with the emerging twentieth-century stress on human experience.

While League leaders herald the naturalness of breast feeding, they emphasize that it is not only an instinct but one that needs to be shaped and cultivated. The League's most important teaching tool is the mother-to-mother sharing of experiences. In other words, the women of La Leche League strive to employ both divine design and rational choice as sources for the "natural" principles of obligation that guide good mothering through breast feeding. This reliance on the natural is inappropriate not only because it has inherent ambiguities but also because it mis-colors the League's relationship to the scientific community. The League acknowledges a great debt to the scientific community, yet it often uses "nature" and its cognates as weapons against those members of the scientific community with whom it disagrees. More recently, overtly religious language about the naturalness of breast feeding has appeared less frequently in League literature. In spite of this semantic shift, breast feeding as a natural way to good mothering and a continued emphasis on the natural differences between mothering and fathering remain League beliefs. On the other hand, League author Dorothy Brewster maintains that every breast-feeding situation is atypical and that "normal" is whatever works best for each unique breast-feeding couple.[26]

La Leche League need not abandon breast feeding's naturalness as a guiding principle if that principle is put within the context of a coherent strategy for mothering in the contemporary world. This strategy begins by acknowledging that the sociobiological tendencies and needs inherent in the dependent-infant–adult-as-caretaker situation are not moral values but "premoral" ones. They are among the many values from which human beings must choose. It must also be acknowledged that problems in practical moral reasoning will appear if one premoral good is given priority so far above all others that any objectivity is lost. Breast feeding can be a good decision, but it does not render the mother who so chooses a moral human being. Rather, breast feeding is among those goods that prospective parents consider but may not be able to realize. Decisions about infant nurturance move into the arena of moral choice after they have been weighed with other premoral possibilities. At this point, the virtuous parent attempts to maximize premoral goods over premoral evils. Sometimes this maximizing is easy to discern. It could happen that the economic well-being of other family members calls for bottle-feeding the new infant. On the other hand, economic sacrifice may be required if the infant thrives only on human milk. Most of the time, prospective parents confront cloudier choices such as a mother's desire for more freedom or a father's wish to participate in every aspect of infant care. La Leche League plays an important role at this juncture. For those parents who seek its help, the League offers scientific facts, counseling, and inspired narrative to help mothers and fathers determine a course of action.

La Leche League's wealth of information, goodwill, and experience can aid parents in moving past the arena of premoral choices to the action that is the right one in their situation. This is the action that really does maximize the premoral good and minimize the premoral evil. This is the choice that activates the morally good. Other choices may be well intended but fail to activate true moral value.

The League's firm conviction that breast feeding is naturally good can be translated to mean that it ranks high among the biological premoral goods. This conviction gains strength through the League approach. The association communicates not primarily through its published literature but through its group meetings and through mother-to-mother phone counseling. This system allows League leaders to individualize their assistance to mother-infant dyads. Leaders take the time to understand the unique challenges each mother confronts. At the same time, their firm belief that the breast-feeding relationship ought to be maximized to the fullest extent possible means that they are unlikely to turn to artificial feeding unnecessarily. This contrasts with well-intended medical advice that fails the moral enterprise by placing an infant on a formula that will not fully meet his or her needs, even though the situation did not require this action. Dr. Jack Newman, a Canadian pediatrician who has published widely on breast feeding and is the founder of the breast-feeding clinic at the Hospital for Sick Children in Toronto, notes that even the most well-meaning physicians lack the time that a League counselor can give to a breast-feeding challenge.[27]

The League leader yearns not just to be correct but to contribute to the flourishing of the good. She desires that her encounters with new mothers will make their world a better place. In her keynote address to the Fourteenth International Conference, Edwina Froehlich declared that parenting not only requires but develops virtue so that, when a person has raised a child, one is a more virtuous person.[28] Today's League leaders may not speak, as the founders did, of breast feeding as part of the world that God has made, but they do emphasize that breast feeding belongs to the *real* world. Author and League leader Tine Thevenin claims that the differences in mothering versus fathering approaches toward an infant are differences not of choice but of design. For Thevenin, research in both cultural anthropology and biology bears witness that gender differences in parenting are in the best interest of all family members.[29] As such, it is a value to be protected. Even though "God" language is avoided in official League literature, during her talk at the Fourteenth International Conference, Thevenin unhesitatingly claimed that mothers' instincts and tendencies toward nurturing and connectedness are "natural" and "God-given." Thus, although the leaders of the 1990s may not perceive any tie with the religious past of the League's founders, they have inherited those women's strong moral convictions. Anwar Fazal, chairperson of the World Alliance for Breastfeeding Action, envisioned the bottle- versus breast-feeding "battle" as one between "greed" and "love." According to Fazal, "The reality of the world today is that we are combating a 'triangle of evil,' composed of the technology of violence, the international business monopolies, and waste." She urges, "We need to counter this with a 'triangle of care,' composed of balance and harmony, understanding, and accountability. There is no question that La Leche League is engaged in a moral struggle. We are dealing with monsters [the formula companies] who throw babies into the river to drown."[30] Convictions such as these are rooted in League beliefs that the world as they see it is "God's world." This moral viewpoint lacks the realization that existential anxiety functions in all humans no matter how good or bad the parenting they receive has been.

THE HEART AND SOUL OF "LLLOVE"

La Leche League leaders often speak of the psychological need for love. Those who have been well loved, they believe, love well. The League approach to infant care influences not only its vision of women's nature but also its understanding of the dynamics of love within the family. Within this belief exists an adherence to gender-specific definitions of loving.

According to Brenda Hunter, a psychologist and speaker at the La Leche League Fourteenth International Conference in 1995, humans need both a mother's and a father's love. We need a mother's consistent, responsive love, and from our fathers we need love that protects and teaches competency. Hunter maintained that, for women, growing up loved is essential, because women are the "intimacy experts" of the family.[31] She also emphasized that a baby's greatest need for his or her mother's love is from birth to eighteen months. She upheld the principle that only the briefest separations are acceptable if the mother wants to give her infant the best possible foundation in feeling loved and learning to love. Critical reflection on these statements reveals that Hunter has conflated the concept of health with a concept of moral obligation. In doing so, she offers both a theory of virtue, love as the central dynamic of family life, and a general principle of obligation, mother-infant proximity.

This principle of obligation can sometimes appear to revolve around a mother who sacrifices herself as a unique person in order to meet the needs of other family members. League members, however, deny that devotion to family means self-sacrifice. Being invested in their children is valued by these mothers. It is understood as a self-evident good, that is, something considered morally good as a matter of natural motivation. For La Leche League mothers, breast feeding is an important moment of self-actualization as well as a basic natural need of their infants. Examining the meaning of love as mutuality in League thought, a meaning that closely resembles some Catholic interpretations of neighbor love, illuminates the experiential reality of these avowals. At the same time, while the League's ethic of nurturing may be compatible with a Catholic Christian ethic of neighbor love, it is also in tension with it.

The League's understanding of love as mutuality closely resembles Stephen Pope's proposed "order of love" for Catholic ethics. According to Pope, Thomas Aquinas rejected the Augustinian insistence that Christian love requires that we feel the same level of regard for all persons. Aquinas advocated the principle that both charity, which is an inclination of grace, and natural affection, which is the inclination of nature, flow from divine wisdom. Aquinas was aware that Jesus apparently rejected the primacy of blood loyalty, and he interpreted this to mean not that natural affection ought to be neutralized but that a distinction needs to be made between ordered and disordered love. For Aquinas charity actually escalates, refines, and magnifies rather than demolishes or forsakes the moral virtues that govern domestic love and justice. Thus, God orders human love through our inborn tendencies, including our biological ones.[32]

For La Leche League mothers, when the "neighbor" of neighbor love is a family member, especially an infant or small child, "love your neighbor as yourself" becomes "in loving your neighbor you are loving yourself." Mary Ann Cahill described the baby as a most generous little soul, ready to give his or her heart. As the mother gives of herself, the baby responds with a gift of love that enriches the mother. It is a reciprocal giving.[33]

A serious weakness in Aquinas's understanding of the natural law was his reliance on the available Aristotelian biology and its narrow perspective. Pope advanced sociobiology as a more accurate source to aid in the understanding of the ordering of love. From a sociobiological point of view, human love flows from millions of years of hominoid evolution. It must be seen as standing within the context of a vast evolutionary framework. Human affective and social capacities are the natural outgrowth of the shaping influence of natural selection.[34] La Leche League comprehends this interaction of biology with affective and social capacities. League mothers believe that breast feeding is not only the biologically optimal choice but also a pleasurable and self-actualizing experience that strengthens their sense of self and contributes to their ability to become socially active persons who work for the good of the community. There are numerous examples of League women using the principles that they acquired as members to enhance other activist efforts. For example, several members joined the September 26, 1990, candlelight vigil across the street from United Nations headquarters during the international conference on the Year of the Child. League mothers sat beneath a banner that read, "Breastfeeding: The World's Greatest Natural Resource." One leader who was present later wrote, "I suddenly had a small understanding of what this was. I realized that when people join together for the welfare of all, something changes. Our world can change, but the change begins in our minds and hearts."[35]

Mother-infant reciprocity is a central principle of the League's understanding of the meaning of love. The League's principle of mutuality, however, extends beyond the mother-infant dyad in many ways. When the women of La Leche League carry their nurturing message beyond their family confines, they are extending "LLLove" to families who ask for help.

Pope held that when family bonds were secure, this created the emotional basis for an expansive love for persons outside the family. Intrafamilial love becomes a central locus of the ethics of love. Sociobiology's theories of kin altruism and of reciprocity stress the human tendency to focus care on our blood relatives before others and to order this care according to the closeness of the blood tie. Pope believed this outlook highlights "important features of social life and morality that need to be respected and promoted within an ethics of love." Kin altruism accents the inner tension caused by conflicting claims made by "various objects of affection and loyalty."[36] It underscores the imperfect choices that we are required to make when loyalties are irreconcilable. League mothers order their loving carefully within and without the family. The needs of infants come first. Even when other family concerns cause difficulties in meeting the needs of infants, League mothers evolve complex strategies to uphold this principle. They strongly believe that a reciprocal relationship exists not only between the mother and the baby but also between the mother-infant dyad and other family members.

We must be cautious when depending on sociobiological theories. Reductionism and materialism plague them. Many aspects of human life are not open to biological explanation. Humans are intersubjective and loyal and affective in ways that supersede strictly biological bonds. Personal, cultural, and economic forces are other important factors that help us form human bonds.

La Leche League lacks the critical self-awareness to give these other factors due consideration. The association promotes breast feeding across cultures as every mother and child's right, because it understands breast feeding to be biologically and psychologically superior to artificial infant feeding. Throughout its existence the League's basic premise has remained the same. All babies have an inherent right to their mother's milk. Pediatrician and League supporter Dr. Linda Black promoted faith in nature's wisdom and urged maternal outrage in the face of the widespread loss of breast feeding. Although she conceded that breast feeding is a culturally rooted experience, she conflated the twentieth-century Western experience with all other such experiences. She claimed that it ought to be a cultural fact that women receive their breast-feeding help from a circle of supportive, experienced women. Doctors, she warned, have to be careful not to take breast feeding away from the mother. She cautioned, "We doctors need to walk softly around this ancient rite."[37]

Recently the League has begun to listen more closely to the women of other cultures. In such cultures, especially in developing areas of the world, the League approach to promoting breast feeding can be counterproductive. In addition, League leaders are more aware that, as Black acknowledged in her presentation, "sometimes breastfeeding should not work and it doesn't; sometimes it should work and it doesn't; some mothers won't breastfeed, some babies won't nurse."[38] More such open statements of the limits of La Leche League ideology are needed to guide the League in its further growth.

chapter 9

· ·

Coping Strategies for a
Changing Environment

La Leche League continues to grow. Its members exert an ever-expanding influence in the area of infant nutrition. Are they going to be as effective as they hope? Are there changes that the League could make that would strengthen its chances of remaining an important voice in family advocacy?

In a 1991 study, sociologist Florence Andrews proposed that the central characteristic of La Leche League is behavioral control through sanctions that are either inferred or explicitly articulated. She believed that, whereas the League's basic philosophy once flourished in a nurturing environment, that environment has eroded over the period of its existence. Thus, Andrews advanced the theory that League mothers have modified their approach and their beliefs to accommodate pressures from a changing society. Andrews concluded, "As contradictions between League practices and social arrangements in the larger society have become sharper, the coping strategies of the organization have been directed toward articulating, revising, or extending those aspects which need clarification — those which are subject to the most threatening attack."[1]

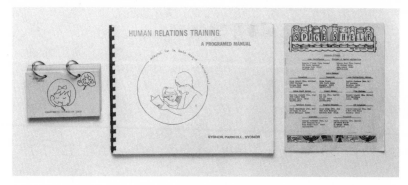

Because the leader is the all-important connection between the new mother and the League, as well as the League's liaison with the broader community, leader training is a slow, careful process accompanied by its own set of publications. The League also keeps leaders in touch with one another through state newsletters such as Illinois's *Spice Shelf*.

Two facets of Andrews's perception of La Leche League do not adhere with the actual praxis of the League. First, the League was not founded within a nurturing environment. From its inception, the association has had to cope with an unsupportive culture. When the League was begun, bottle feeding was the prevailing means of infant nurturance, and mothers were expected to attend to male experts on child care. Soon after the founding of the League, members of the association were advised to curb religious language in references to breast feeding so that the surrounding secular culture would not misunderstand their purpose. In reality, the only League ideal that conformed to the prevailing culture was the belief that mothers and children needed to be together. This aspect of the association's philosophy has been articulate, extensive, and clear.

Second, the major characteristic of La Leche League is not control but dialectical conversation. League leaders are not only articulate teachers, they are attentive listeners. In fact, they listen much more than they talk. League philosophy and practice have expanded the organization's scope and renewed its promise not in defense against a perceived attack but in response to new ways of thinking and doing that have been presented to it. Just as individual leaders shape meetings into constructive dialogue with other mothers, so does the association as a whole engage in dialectical encounters with its ongoing conversation partners: medical science, feminism, and religious ethics.

LA LECHE LEAGUE'S GROWING
PARTNERSHIP WITH MEDICINE

When La Leche League first introduced physicians' seminars into its program, its leaders were aware that doctors knew the advantages of breast feeding. What they sought to communicate to doctors and other health professionals was that knowing the advantages of breast feeding was not enough.

Linda Black observed that the gap between physicians' acknowledgment of breast milk's superiority and the reality of their care of the mother-infant dyad goes back to the nineteenth century. At that time, doctors caring for infants were confronting an infant mortality rate that was between 30 and 50 percent. While doctors knew that breast-fed babies did better, they considered mothers who did not succeed at breast feeding as "flawed."[2] Doctors believed mothers were losing the breast-feeding instinct as well as their other womanly instincts. Jack Newman has noted two other false notions that have hampered the ability of physicians to support breast feeding universally. One was the idea that a "cultured" woman could not breast-feed. A second false notion was that the nearer "to nature" a woman lived, the more "normal" her milk would be.[3] According to Black, the doctors had so little insight into the reasons women failed at breast feeding that they felt unable to advise breast feeding for the infants under their care. Therefore, they suggested artificial feeding as the safer choice.

Challenged by the medical world's discouraging attitude toward breast feeding, La Leche League strives to demonstrate that the hindrances to successful breast feeding are far more complicated than a woman's social status or her cultural background. League mothers have taken on the formidable task of engaging health professionals as partners in the care and nutrition of infants and young children. According to Newman, "Teamwork with lay persons is difficult for health professionals." Most health professionals are products of bottle-feeding societies. For them, "scientific" infant feeding is much more comforting. They tend to believe that what cannot be measured cannot be known. In the process of their education, physicians do not learn about the joy of suckling because observations of mothers and babies actually nursing are rare. Physicians are scientists who are rarely touched by the poetry of breast feeding. Progress is a deeply seated faith principle of medicine. Since breast milk cannot be "made better," it lacks scientific appeal.[4]

Despite these difficulties, the partnership between health professionals and La Leche League has grown. The dialogue between them has flourished because League leaders have extended their nurturing to the physicians with whom they have worked. This has been accomplished in several ways. First, the League respects the limits of its expertise and communicates this to the medical world. Second, a partnership with League leaders offers physicians a way of overcoming the overwhelming time limits of their practice. Ameliorating a breast-feeding problem sometimes takes hours, even days, of counseling. League leaders communicate to physicians that they have the time to spend that doctors often lack. Third, League leaders are cultivating doctors who support breast feeding. They send mothers to them. They follow up with positive feedback about individual mothers' positive experiences. Fourth, the League informs its leaders about anti-breast-feeding studies that physicians receive so that when a leader approaches a doctor she is ready to offer her counterarguments respectfully. Many times she can also point out that the study was sponsored by a formula company.

Many doctors have responded in kind. Because the League's work and its concepts have received international professional recognition, many individual physicians are choosing to explain the differences between breast milk and artificial formula to their patients. Doctors are learning to think of telling mothers about these differences as "informed consent." They are learning to see their true role over the course of the *normal* breast-feeding situation as offering information and encouragement, not management. Dr. Gary Freed sought to unravel the dilemma presented by the contradiction that, although breast feeding had received highest recommendations from medical organizations for three decades, by the late 1980s the incidence of breast feeding was decreasing. He discovered that many physicians did not consider breast-feeding counseling worthy of their time. They tended to refer all breast-feeding mothers to lactation consultants or nurses. It is the doctor, however, not the in-hospital consultants, who sees the mother before the birth and does follow-up care. Thus, it is the physician who will have the most impact on women and their infants. Unfortunately, Freed's findings also revealed that these same physicians were woefully lacking in proper breast-feeding information. He suggested that the solution would be more and better breast-feeding education during medical training.[5]

Other health professionals, recognizing their own areas of ignorance, refer mothers with problems to someone who can help with breast feeding after the mother leaves the hospital. They no longer simply put the baby on a bottle. Thus, the dialogical nature of the conversation between La Leche League and medical science contributes to our understanding of the premoral goods that compose a healthy family life. The task that both the League and the medical world still need to undertake is to recognize that they are engaged in an ethical endeavor. A joint affirmation of the value of breast feeding entails an acceptance of the practice as a premoral good that must be balanced with other premoral goods. Consequently, the moral responsibility set before them is that of ordering the breast-feeding relationship within the myriad of family realities. Families everywhere would be the beneficiaries of the recognition of the ethical facets of this dialogue. Nevertheless, although the League speaks of introducing physicians to the "poetry of breast feeding" and doctors call for revering "this ancient women's rite," neither group is yet inviting ethicists to the conversation table.

A BROADENED UNDERSTANDING
OF THE ROLE OF WOMEN

Recent feminist thought has recognized that feminism is multidimensional. Three aspects of this discovery are particularly important in the dialogue between La Leche League and feminism.

First, women are beginning to resist being pitted against one another on the basis of the choices they make when they become mothers. Betty Friedan recently insisted that being a feminist does not mean a woman has to be employed outside the home. She affirmed that feminism seeks first of all to ensure that women have real choices. This quest means feminists are giving new importance to women's traditional contributions and to a new integration of family and home with work.[6] Such claims reflect a new appreciation for the complex moral choices families face and a new opportunity to discover an ethical ordering of premoral goods within the family. Also, as Miller-McLemore insists, the good of the family relies on the deep concern of nonparental members of society as well.

At the global level, Third World feminists are calling for a critique of "neoliberal" feminism. These women stress that an assumption of universality is false because it blinds women to their differences. This dangerous oversight permits women of the former colonial powers to ignore the reality that they are not only victims but also oppressors.

Finally, as Janet Sayers has noted, "Biology — *as it interacts with socioeconomic and historical factors* — directly affects women's experience and how they live roles within the social order."[7] It reduces the importance of the way individual women experience their differences from individual men. Mothering is different from fathering because the experience of motherhood begins with pregnancy, childbirth, and nursing, which cannot be directly experienced by men. While mothers differ enormously in the range of their responses to their infants, most women experience more intense feelings toward their babies than do men. A recent study reveals that even when both parents in a family identified themselves as the primary caretaker, the mothers spent more time than did the fathers worrying about their children when separated from them. Fathers found separation less distracting and easier to endure than did their wives. These women, many of them professionals, often felt so closely connected to their infants that they could not meaningfully make a choice to pursue their career with "fast-track" dedication. Several other studies have demonstrated that it is not only feelings that identify the mother as the more attached parent. Various realities of domestic life, whether in one- or two-income families, all point toward a greater involvement by mothers than fathers in most child-care situations. Despite this fact, there has been a silence about maternal feelings, with a resulting unnecessary cost to families. University of Chicago Law School professor Mary Becker believes that women must overcome their fear of a charge of essentialist thinking. Unless maternal feelings are explored openly, society faces the unnecessary emotional cost of inappropriate separation for both children and mothers. Being silent about maternal feelings has not resulted in equality in marriage. Nor has equalized parenting ended women's subordination to men. Therefore, Becker holds, women may need to question whether equal parenting should be a primary goal. In the meantime, she asserts, we must base our actions on the known emotional needs of women and children.[8] Yet it remains appropriate that our society should strive to create more equalitarian families. This calls for an immensely altered socialization process for boys and girls. But, at this time, it appears best to respect the emotional needs of mothers and infants by structuring optimum mother-baby closeness into society's expectations of the family.

La Leche League enters into dialogue with feminism at all three points. First, the League praxis has grown gradually more open to the needs of the employed mother while remaining supportive of the at-home mother. Recent publications by the League demonstrate a new sensitivity to contemporary mothers and the variety of their actual challenges. Both *New Beginnings*, the League journal for breast-feeding parents, and *Leaven*, the newsletter for leaders, carry an increasing number of narratives about mothers who successfully combine breast feeding with employment outside the home. Also, more and more stories are appearing about husbands whose coparenting includes spending more time than their wives in actual hands-on child care. The League's most thorough exploration of both subjects is Kaye Lowman's *Of Cradles and Careers*. Lowman, a League administrator, has been a member of La Leche League for twenty-five years. Her comprehensive book includes research on flexible working arrangements and other part-time job opportunities. It illustrates each point with personal stories and photos from career women/mothers who are, according to Lowman, revolutionizing the workplace.

Second, La Leche League has increasingly included mothers from developing nations at its conferences. The critique that these mothers have sometimes leveled at the League's "Western" approach has been taken seriously. The League's Fourteenth International Conference included a three-session track entitled "The Establishment of Mother-to-Mother Support in Economically Disadvantaged and Low-Literate Communities in Developing Areas of the World." During these sessions, mothers from several South American countries, Malaysia, the Philippines, the Caribbean islands, and several African nations gathered to describe mother-to-mother support within the context of their various cultures. Their first goal was to give mother-to-mother support a definition that included shared principles within a spirit of multiculturalism. Using both small- and large-group discussions, the mothers created a definition that reflected the best gains of feminism without contradicting the goals of La Leche League. The definition reads, "Mother-to-mother support is experienced mothers offering culturally sensitive information to other mothers who seek a rewarding breastfeeding experience. Experienced mothers aim to establish a relationship of trust and respect. Together with the new mother, they explore options that allow these mothers to meet their own challenges and make their own decisions. This method of support empowers mothers by giving them a feeling of self-realization."

While participants in these sessions did not articulate a specifically feminist agenda, their discussion revealed an awareness of the unique feminist issues that confront women in developing countries. Among them was the degree to which male dominance prevails in these cultures. For instance, when a member of the group that was discussing ways to approach an employer suggested speaking firmly but deferentially about a baby's needs, a leader from India declared this unrealistic. "If the poor mothers in my country speak to an employer about 'their needs,' he would immediately fire them," she claimed. Her words inspired the group to continue working toward a solution that might work in such situations as well as in the face of other entrenched policies. A solution, which brought general consent, was to have the entire mother-to-mother support group approach the employer. This theme of women working together in a very public way for and with other women appeared several times through the three-session track.[9]

Third, La Leche League continues to be a major advocate of the concept that, although both parents are equally important to the child, their roles in child care are neither identical nor easily exchangeable. La Leche League leader and author Tine Thevenin's book, *Mothering and Fathering: The Gender Differences in Child Rearing*, explains this League concept. Thevenin insists that women are the "nurturers" and men are the "encouragers." She holds that, although both parents nurture and encourage, mothers lean toward offering a safe haven and fathers toward pushing the child to achieve. There are, she concedes, a multitude of gradations and variations in this basic structure; however, this does not change the reality that fathers' and mothers' approaches not only are different but also may serve as a source of potential conflict. This is because each parent understands his or her approach as the right one. Neither sees that the approaches are complementary and that both are necessary for the child's healthy development.

These differences, Thevenin claims, are the result of both biology and culture. To ignore them is detrimental not only to children but to their parents as well. Misconceptions can arise when our society does not recognize that male expectations differ from female ones. As an example,

Thevenin cites the fact that, while our society expects women to be the primary caretakers, it also expects them to follow the advice of male "experts." Therefore, within the world of child care we have come to value the male viewpoint that stresses independence over interdependence. This focus obscures the mother's tendency to allow children to mature gradually, allowing dependence as an essential aspect of the human personality.

Many feminists, even those who recognize that socialization has created major differences between male and female approaches to children, might still find Thevenin's claims dangerously essentialist, but critique cannot obscure the important fact that women's ways of knowing and guiding have been undervalued and need to be reintegrated into the cultural norm. Beyond these three issues, both League literature and the sessions at League conferences are devoted to a broadened spectrum of women's issues. They include women's physical and psychological health beyond the area of breast feeding, meeting the challenge of single parenting, grandparenting, and coping with the monetary challenges of a shrinking family income. It is clear that La Leche League represents a principal advocate for women. Consequently, La Leche League praxis, as it is presently evolving, remains open to the new realism in feminist thought.

A PILGRIM PEOPLE ENGAGED
IN DIALOGICAL OUTREACH

Starting with Leo XIII's *Rerum Novarum* (*On the Condition of Workers*), the encyclicals of the Roman Catholic pontiffs have developed a vision of a just society within the social, economic, political, and cultural realities of the age. Certain key themes pervade this teaching. They are the social nature of the human person, the solidarity of the human family, the dignity of work, and the special claim of the poor and the vulnerable.[10]

Since the Second Vatican Council, Catholic encyclical teaching has accommodated the accelerated pace of social change in our contemporary world and has developed unique metaphors to express each of these four key themes. These themes do not encompass all of contemporary Catholic thinking. Peace, for example, is a major theme of Catholic social writing. These four themes do, however, find strong echoes in the writing and practices of La Leche League. Conversely, certain deep metaphors resonate in the League that are either absent or weak in Catholic teaching. The encyclicals since Vatican II express a fresh appreciation for the affective and historical dimensions of human experience. They perceive the historical context as the milieu for the divine-human encounter. The church is envisioned as a pilgrim people engaged in dialogical outreach, inspired by the ever-present dialogical Spirit.[11]

Although no literature is available that would provide an exact parallel between La Leche League's understanding of a just society and that of the Roman Catholic Church, the key themes found in the encyclicals prevail in La Leche League praxis. These key themes also exist in the teachings of many contemporary faith communities. From these roots, they influence the moral sensibilities of the American society.

The deep metaphors of League thought allow it the necessary freedom and the essential self-awareness to actualize its members' core morality. These metaphors have evolved from the need to respond in an open and caring way to the increasing pace of family and cultural life. And, thus, the League can also be envisioned as a pilgrim people engaged in dialogical outreach. Within this outreach again exist the four key themes named above: the social nature of the human person, the solidarity of the human family, the dignity of work, and the special claim of the poor and the vulnerable.

First, both communities share the view that humans are by their nature interrelational. *Gaudium et Spes* (*The Church in the Modern World*) emphasized the individual human as social being, noting that persons are not "isolated, self-directed singularities."[12] This understanding, which so contrasts with liberal individualism, is found throughout League literature. The League's strongest principle, the right of the mother and baby to be together, is based on the conviction that it is necessary not only for the psychological development of the infant but also for the social development of both mother and child. It is this latter inclination that causes many working mothers to choose breast feeding. One mother reports, "Nursing Nicki when I get home is the most relaxing thing I can do. I can't imagine working and not nursing my baby."[13]

Second, both the Catholic Church and La Leche League cherish the solidarity of the human family. After Vatican II, encyclical and episcopal teaching moved away from the notion that Roman Catholicism is necessarily linked to Western civilization. For Catholicism, the entire world of human interrelationships is imbued with God's presence. No area of expertise exists that is outside God's dominion. "Neither politics nor economics, neither national interest nor international affairs, neither technology nor commerce, neither aesthetics nor productivity, can ultimately be a law unto itself."[14]

La Leche League's many programs designed to reach out to impoverished mothers and to women in developing nations reflect this same conviction. Sociologist Maryanne Locklin studied the League's peer counselor program, which is designed to initiate breast feeding in the inner cities of the United States. She found that, like the first La Leche League leaders, the peer counselors were knowledgeable, nurturing, and passionate about their mission. They do far more than offer breast-feeding advice. They call their clients frequently and encourage new mothers to call them at any time of the day or night. They provide mothers with self-esteem, inner strength, and a sense of purpose in their lives.[15]

Third, the dignity of work is a central tenet of both twentieth-century Catholic teaching and of La Leche League practice. The leaders of Catholicism understand Christian teaching to include a "gospel of work." Work's effect on the dignity of the worker takes precedence over the objective goal of the work activity. This "humanization" of work counteracts the market's bifurcation of persons into consumers and workers. John Paul II argued that "the basis for determining the value of human work is not primarily the kind of work being done, but the fact that the one who is doing it is a person."[16] Robert Kuttner, an economics journalist, sees several ways the Catholic perspective serves as a counterweight to the claims that laissez-faire individualism is necessary economics. First of all, programs that integrate the work with nonwork aspects of human life, such as parental leaves, make it possible for humans to be workers without sacrificing their dedication to other human pursuits. Second, Catholic social thought functions in America as an effective opponent to the claims of pure capitalism. Kuttner claims one need not be Catholic to "appreciate that a social conception of the market also makes for a more sustainable and dynamic capitalism."[17]

Women's place within this "gospel of work" has been unique. Beginning with the midcentury, Catholic teaching began to assume the need to educate young women both for marriage and motherhood and for a career. The belief that women's female uniqueness would enable them to use their education to change the world into a more hospitable environment fueled these efforts. More recently, John Paul II called for a recognition of the dignity due to women working within and without the home. He did so, however, in language that warned that women should "fulfill their tasks in accordance with their own nature" without having to abandon "what is specific to them and at the expense of the family in which women as mothers have an irreplaceable role."[18] Whereas such a warning can be read to be an attempt to reassert that a woman's primary place is at home, it can also be understood to say that each woman must find her own specific way of balancing her roles within and outside the family.

The founding mothers of La Leche League flourished within a Catholic milieu that encouraged women to think of themselves as both homemakers and world shakers. The enthusiasm generated by this conviction infused the fledgling organization with a commitment to maintaining the dignity of women's work. Presented from the late sixties with a challenge to the dignity of homemaking, La Leche League's greatest efforts have been directed at preserving the dignity of work within the home. Founder Mary Ann Cahill contends that she knows no one who would turn back the clock to the seemingly simpler though much more limited era when the home was the special domain of women, a domain that some women felt offered them considerable freedom although others found it stifling. She and other leaders, however, have found over their years of counseling that several factors motivate women to choose the role of homemaker. The League works to support these women and to uphold the dignity of their choice. It can be a courageous decision. Returning to the comfortable, familiar routine of a well-liked job can seem the more reassuring choice. Being a mother is a unique experience, one it is impossible for a woman to know beforehand. Faced with uncertainty about her ability to mother well, which contrasts with the confidence she feels in the workplace, a first-time mother may elect to leave her baby with an experienced child-care worker. Further, the mother may worry that staying at home will cut her off from the broader community. League mothers offer themselves as a small supportive community that allows women to extend the scope of being at-home mothers. They encourage women to transform their former social patterns based on their employment network to one that includes other at-home mothers engaged in community-related activities. Keeping in touch with their professional field is another way League mothers stay involved in the world beyond the home. They continue to read trade journals and recently published books about advances or debates in their professional areas. When an infant no longer needs full-time care, they enroll in courses in local universities. Many women remain concerned that years at home will hamper their future reentry into the workplace. Cahill admits that there are no guarantees, although she points out that even for people who have always been employed, "job security is a tenuous thing at best."[19]

La Leche League literature emphasizes that the mother who remains at home to care for her children need not assume that this decision confers on her the role of sole housekeeper. The League resists the notion that husbands who provide the full financial support of the family need not contribute to maintaining the home. From an alternative perspective, many League mothers are comfortable with doing whatever amount of housework is possible while giving priority to their children's needs. These mothers assert that their efforts render their homes more pleasant for all and allow the whole family relaxed and companionable evenings and weekends. All these factors — support for the new mothers, encouragement for involvement in the broader community, and respect for homemaking — demonstrate that La Leche League beliefs resound with the theme of the dignity of work.

In its response to the new realism in feminist thought, the League demonstrates its support of the dignity of women's work outside the home as well. In this the League's stance contrasts with some encyclical teaching. Amata Miller of the National Catholic Social Justice Lobby notes that in *Centesimus Annus* (*One Hundred Years*) John Paul II missed an opportunity to address a critical justice issue. Because the pope defines "just wages" as those that allow a man to support his family, he ignores that a majority of women who work outside the home do so to support their families.[20]

The fourth key issue is the special claim of the poor and the vulnerable to our care. Many twentieth-century Catholic writers, leaders, and teachers have recognized that until recently the original Christian orientation to the needs of the poor was muted by the church's stake in the established order. Beginning with Leo XIII's *On the Condition of Workers*, an evolution has occurred in the church's awareness that God sides with the poor. Leo demanded that the wealthy, the employers, and the state respond in charity to the impoverished state of workers. In his *Quadra-*

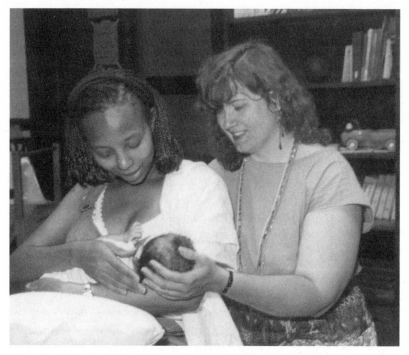

La Leche League takes its breast-feeding curriculum into high schools, helping teen mothers develop a positive self-image and parenting skills through breast feeding their infants.

gesimo Anno (*The Reconstruction of the Social Order*), Pius XI advocated activism for social change as a primary Christian vocation. John XXIII shifted the focus to the urgency of alleviating world poverty. The bishops of Vatican II echoed this theme, naming response to the poor as central to discipleship. Paul VI built on this teaching. In 1967, recognizing the overwhelming reality of world poverty, he urged all-encompassing trans- formations of existing social structures. The following year, at Medellín, the Latin American bishops applied these teachings to their continent. They committed themselves to enabling the poor to effect their own liberation. John Paul II has continually reaffirmed that care for the poor is a central Christian principle. In their pastoral letters, the bishops of the United States have also developed the theme that Christians must accept the responsibility that concern for the poor is their most urgent moral priority. When Christians undertake their vocation to commit to making working with the poor a focus of their discipleship, they transform their lives in several ways. Employers and managers give labor priority over capital. They pay wages that allow workers to both provide an adequate level of living and save against future setbacks. Individuals and families simplify their lifestyles, consuming less and sharing goods, expertise, and knowledge. State officials respond to their nation's call to organize the government to protect rights and provide for the poor. Church members, hierarchy and laity alike, bring all peoples into their community. Catholic Christians also accept that each one is responsible for a share in the world's injustice. They recognize their need for a conversion to a life of justice. They integrate faith and action by taking part in public life so as to transform corporate and governmental structures from within.

La Leche League praxis is by its nature devoted to those whom League members perceive as the most vulnerable members of our society, newborn infants and young children and their mothers. League women view the modern culture as having created "a situation which is having a profound effect on our society from the macroeconomic level of a squandered natural resource to the individual misery of a sick child or a confused, unhappy woman." League members worry lest "in all the struggle for economic and sexual justice a baby's needs are often neglected and, during this crucial phase of physical and emotional development, many are damaged for ever."[21] League members feel called to transform this unjust situation into one of justice and caring. The League's earliest efforts focused on helping the individual mother with breast-feeding problems.

While continuing to focus on individual mothers and their needs, League members have joined forces with others who work for better conditions for mothers and babies in a multitude of situations. For example, they have joined with others to protest the exclusion of the breast-feeding mother from the workplace. They recognize that what should be solved through rational negotiations becomes instead an agonizing decision for the mother who needs to remain employed. This recognition has motivated the League to engage the corporate world in dialogue. Both individual mothers and the League's highest-level leaders are working to redefine the American work ethic. This includes helping each woman find her unique balance between work and family and working to bring about more baby-friendly workplaces. This is an ongoing endeavor. The attitude persists that motherhood belongs in private places. Both business persons and the public in general continue to view the integration of mothers and babies into public life with ridicule and alarm. Mothers continue to make more compromises than do their employers.

The League's outreach to the vulnerable goes beyond the babies and mothers caught in the whirling currents of the American workplace. Identifying teenage pregnancy as a reality that must be faced, not ignored, the League has taken its breast-feeding curriculum into some high schools. This course work has had a profound effect on the girls who have attended the classes. They have come to realize that a woman's readiness for motherhood is invariably linked to her commitment to be present with her baby on an ongoing basis. These girls come to accept that, if they cannot handle the responsibility of being a consistent nurturer in a child's life, they are not ready to conceive a baby.[22]

The League's work in the developing areas of the world is another example of its commitment to the poor and the vulnerable. League members realize that as women who have some measure of power or influence, however small, they must recognize the enormous contribution that millions of oppressed women in traditional roles make to human prosperity and welfare by breast feeding their infants and toddlers.

Ava Wilhite Navin, a Guatemalan mother, asserts, "The League's message is especially important in a developing country like Guatemala, where the nutritional status of children deteriorates as soon as they are weaned. Traditional practices give way too readily to the 'modern' ways of bottles (impossible to keep clean) and formula (impossible to afford)."[23]

The League also works with local health agencies. In 1982 the Ministry of Health of Honduras launched an intensive and successful attempt to reverse its country's trend away from breast feeding. Through community education and hospital staff training, the program encouraged Honduran mothers to initiate breast feeding and to extend the number of months they breast-feed. The seven-year project, called Proyecto de Apoyo a la Lactancia Materno, continues to have an impact because of the "outreach efforts which have gotten under way through community support groups organized by La Leche League/Honduras."[24]

Western leaders are learning from mothers and leaders from developing areas that middle-class American solutions will not necessarily work everywhere. At the same time, they are learning that solutions achieved by mothers in the developing areas are often applicable to the dilemmas faced by mothers in their local areas. United States leaders are renewed by the passionate advocacy of women such as Anwar Fazal, an Indian physician, who proclaimed with conviction that there is "no question that La Leche League is engaged in a moral struggle. We are dealing with monsters who throw babies into the river to drown."[25] A clear statement of a preferential option for the oppressed and the poor, Fazal's call to action expressed the League's increasing awareness of the full scope of its mission.

BEGIN WITH THE MOTHERS

Soon after the League's inception, Herbert Ratner, its "midwife," became aware that the association needed to engage in reflective action in order to achieve its goals. That initial reflection has grounded the further developments in the League praxis. The League's original goal, good mothering through breast feeding, has grown to become a comprehensive ideology of family life. This ideology is richly grounded in multidimensional religioethical metaphors. Such grounding allows the League to continue as a source of family and community renewal and revitalization. In 1981, Ratner expressed his persistent faith that the League would play a major role in turning the already universal medical approval of breast feeding to an actual universal practice. To express his conviction, he cited Jean-Jacques Rousseau: "Would you restore all to their primal duties, begin with the mothers; the results will surprise you."[26]

notes

· ·

INTRODUCTION

1. Herbert Ratner, foreword to La Leche League International, *Womanly Art of Breastfeeding*, 2d ed., vi.

2. Browning, *Religious Thought and the Modern Psychologies*, 9.

CHAPTER 1

1. Except where noted otherwise, this history of La Leche League is based on six sources: the three editions of the La Leche League manual, *The Womanly Art of Breastfeeding*; the 1977 history of the League by Kaye Lowman, *The LLLove Story*; a dialogue between Dr. Herbert Ratner and the founders, published in October 1981 in *Child and Family*; and a series of dialogues between the author and the founders of the League, which took place in March 1993. The manuals and Lowman's book were published by La Leche League International. These sources are detailed in the bibliography but are listed in the notes only in the case of direct quotes.

2. La Leche League International, *Why Nurse Your Baby?*, 3.

3. Founding Mothers, *La Leche League Dialogue*, 5. On March 27, 1958, Dr. Ratner joined with the founding mothers to discuss the purpose of La Leche League. As he expressed it, "In this dialogue, the moderator emulated, to the extent his talents made possible, the Socratic midwife immortalized by Plato." Dr. Ratner's goal was to help the founding mothers determine whether the ideas they taught in the League were true to their own beliefs and grounded "on the realities of Nature." (The discussion was recorded by Caroline E. Ward, the Public Health Educator of Oak Park, Illinois, and was transcribed by Dr. Ratner's secretary, Ruth Uteritz. It was originally published in *Child and Family* 13, nos. 3–4 [1974], and 14, no. 1 [1975].)

4. Founding Mothers, *La Leche League Dialogue*, 5.

5. Apple, *Mothers and Medicine*, 124–25.

6. Lowman, *The LLLove Story*, 14.

7. La Leche League International, *Statement of Policy*.

8. E. M. B., "Mothers and Nursing Don't Always Mix," 3.

9. La Leche League chose to refer to the baby with a masculine pronoun. "We appreciate and applaud the fact that babies come in two genders, male and female, delightful he's and charming she's, . . . we refer to baby only as 'he,' not with sexist intent, but simply for clarity's sake. Mother is unquestionably 'she.'" La Leche League International, *Womanly Art of Breastfeeding*, 3d ed., xvi.

10. Apple, *Mothers and Medicine*, 97.

11. Frisbie, "La Leche League," 21.

12. In this article, Newton cites a 1965 study by John Nash as the source of her information. See Nash, "The Father in Contemporary Culture and Current Psychological Literature," 261–97. Nash's article contains a review of several studies conducted between 1930 and 1965 on the father-child relationship. In it, Nash concludes, "The relative neglect of the father may have distorted our understanding of the dynamics of development and have adversely affected the rearing of males" (262).

13. Beverly Bush Smith, "She Begins Nursing Baby at 11 Weeks to Save Him!," *Chicago Tribune*, August 14, 1960, sec. 5, p. 1.

14. Derrick B. Jelliffe, foreword to Brewster, *You Can Breastfeed Your Baby*, xviii.

15. Founding Mothers, *La Leche League Dialogue*, 20–22.

16. Tompson, "Note to the Reader," 2.

17. Brewster, *You Can Breastfeed Your Baby*, xxvii.

18. "From the Editor," 2.

19. La Leche League of Illinois, "Working with a Leader Applicant," 3.

20. La Leche League International, "Evaluation Form."

21. Barbara King, Franklin Park, Ill., letter to Jule Ward, March 25, 1980.

22. Jule Ward, Chicago, letter to Barbara King, n.d.

23. La Leche League International, "A Special Letter to League Mothers," 1.

24. La Leche League of Ohio, "Some Reminders," 4.

25. Fahey, "Benefits of Being a Leader," 26.

26. Founding Mothers, *La Leche League Dialogue*, 19.

27. Countryman, "New Professional Liaison Department," 27.

28. Kahel and Dyal, *Leader's Handbook*, 28.

29. La Leche League of Maryland and Virginia, [Untitled], n.p.

30. Ruether, *Mary*, 18, 60.

31. "Praxis" as I use it here adheres closely to Thomas Groome's definition of the term as "the consciousness and agency that arise from and are expressed in any and every aspect of people's 'being' as agent-subjects-in-relationship, whether realized in actions that are personal, interpersonal, sociopolitical, or cosmic." See Groome, *Sharing Faith*, 136.

CHAPTER 2

1. Frank, *Persuasion and Healing*, 66.

2. Casebeer, "Who Shall Treat the Children?," 735–43.

3. Apple, *Mothers and Medicine*, 97.

4. Gartner, "Two Thousand Years of Medical Advice on Breast Feeding."

5. Greenley was referring to the *British Medical Journal* of June 12, 1875, which

reported that "during the first month 57 per cent [of infants] die; second month, 21.80 per cent; third month, 15.30 per cent . . . rapidly decreasing as age increases."

6. Greenley, "The Management of Infants under a Year Old," 509–12.

7. Work, "Causes of the Great Mortality in Infancy and Childhood," 618–19.

8. Wood, "Address on Dietetics," 37–39.

9. Apple, *Mothers and Medicine*, 17–18.

10. Rotch, "General Principles Underlying All Good Methods of Infant Feeding," 505.

11. A full discussion of these properties follows in the next chapter.

12. Apple, *Mothers and Medicine*, 23–68.

13. Eley, "Medical Progress," 232.

14. "Editorial: Breast-Fed and Bottle-Fed Babies," 1231–32.

15. Apple, *Mothers and Medicine*, 72–73.

16. Richardson, "How to Nurse Your Baby," 468.

17. Markel and Oski, *H. L. Mencken Baby Book*, 16–17.

18. Spock, *Common Sense Book of Baby and Child Care*, 32–34.

19. Packard, *Human Milk and Infant Formula*, 195.

20. Smith, *Encyclopedia of Baby and Child Care*, 348.

21. Palmer, *Politics of Breastfeeding*, 11.

22. Markel and Oski, *H. L. Mencken Baby Book*, 77.

23. Spock, *Common Sense Book of Baby and Child Care*, 32–33.

24. Boostrom, "Baring the Breast," 414, 416.

25. Jelliffe, "Community and Sociopolitical Considerations of Breastfeeding," 234.

26. Pryor, *Nursing Your Baby*, 4.

27. Newton, *Family Book of Child Care*, 105.

28. Spock, *Common Sense Book of Baby and Child Care*, 33, 37.

29. May, *Better Homes and Gardens Baby Book*, 49.

30. Markel and Oski, *H. L. Mencken Baby Book*, 68.

31. Matson and Kreigh, "They Wanted to Nurse Their Babies," 90.

32. May, *Better Homes and Gardens Baby Book*, 62.

33. Green, *Dr. Green's Baby Book*, 123.

34. Ibid.

35. Spock, *Common Sense Book of Baby and Child Care*, 50, 51.

36. May, *Better Homes and Gardens Baby Book*, 127.

37. Smith, *Encyclopedia of Baby and Child Care*, 376.

38. Palmer, *Politics of Breastfeeding*, 60.

39. Spock, *Common Sense Book of Baby and Child Care*, 16.

40. Ibid., 254–55.

41. Matson and Kreigh, "They Wanted to Nurse Their Babies," 90.

42. "Editorial: Breast-Fed and Bottle-Fed Babies," 1231.

43. Brewster, *You Can Breastfeed Your Baby*, xix.

44. Palmer, *Politics of Breastfeeding*, 38–40.

CHAPTER 3

1. La Leche League International, *Becoming a La Leche League Leader*, n.p.

2. Pryor, *Nursing Your Baby*, 7.

3. Palmer, *Politics of Breastfeeding*, 73–75. Palmer cites Aloià, "Risk Factors for Postmenopausal Osteoporosis," 95–100, and "Nutritional Reviews"; Ing and Pe-

trakis, "Unilateral Breastfeeding and Cancer," 124–27; and Byers, "Lactation and Breast Cancer," 664–73.

4. La Leche League International, *Becoming a La Leche League Leader*.

5. La Leche League International, *Womanly Art of Breastfeeding*, 2d ed., 7.

6. Ibid., 3d ed., 288–92.

7. Ibid., 2d ed., 8.

8. Ibid., 3d ed., 294–96.

9. La Leche League International, *Why Nurse Your Baby?*, n.p.

10. La Leche League International, *Womanly Art of Breastfeeding*, 3d ed., 74–77.

11. Grobman, in *La Leche League News*, 89.

12. Carson, "About Bonding," 89.

13. May, *Better Homes and Gardens Baby Book*, 41.

14. Pryor, *Nursing Your Baby*, 198.

15. Babette Francis, *Journal of Tropical Pediatrics and Environmental Child Health*, quoted without date or page number in La Leche League International, *Womanly Art of Breastfeeding*, 3d ed., 98.

16. Palmer, *Politics of Breastfeeding*, 23–24.

17. Riordan and Auerbach, *Breastfeeding and Human Lactation*, 47.

18. La Leche League International, *Becoming a La Leche League Leader*, n.p.

19. Brewster, *You Can Breastfeed Your Baby*, 150.

20. Ibid., 153–54; La Leche League International, *Womanly Art of Breastfeeding*, 2d ed., 55, 68–69.

21. La Leche League International, *Womanly Art of Breastfeeding*, 3d ed., 126.

22. La Leche League International, *Womanly Art of Breastfeeding*, 1st ed., 17; ibid., 3d ed., 101–2, 159–60.

23. La Leche League International, *Becoming a La Leche League Leader*, n.p.

24. La Leche League International, *Womanly Art of Breastfeeding*, 1st ed., 27.

25. Ibid., 2d ed., 130.

26. Ibid., 130–31.

27. Bonaparte, "Early Weaning," 50.

28. Voyles, "Time to Wean?," 28.

29. La Leche League International, *Womanly Art of Breastfeeding*, 3d ed., 181.

30. Ibid., 182.

31. Ibid., 1st ed., 18.

32. Ibid., 3d ed., 154–55.

33. Spradin, "One and One and Three," 53.

34. La Leche League International, *Womanly Art of Breastfeeding*, 1st ed., 19.

35. Stewart, "A Father Is Born," 42.

36. La Leche League International, *Womanly Art of Breastfeeding*, 2d ed., 116–17.

37. Niles Newton, foreword to La Leche League International, *Womanly Art of Breastfeeding*, 3d ed., xiii.

38. Lisa Sowle Cahill, "Particular Experiences, Shared Goods," in *Sex, Gender, and Christian Ethics*, 15.

CHAPTER 4

1. "Second wave" is a designation given to the feminism that began in Western thought in the early 1960s. This title distinguishes it from the first wave of feminism,

which occurred during the suffrage movement from 1860 to 1920 and lost its major force after women received the vote. Throughout this book, "feminism" refers to the second wave.

2. Tillich, *The Courage to Be*, 151.

3. Degler, *At Odds*, 473.

4. Goldscheider and Waite, *New Families, No Families*, xiii. The resources for their data were the National Longitude Surveys of Labor Market Experience. These surveys each started with five thousand individuals from a wide cross section of Americans. The subjects were followed for at least fifteen years. This allowed them to test the in-depth studies, which provided insight into the "processes underlying behaviors" but whose conclusions were tentative because they included only a small number of individuals (xii).

5. Ibid.

6. Ibid., xiv.

7. Rich, *Of Woman Born*, 29.

8. Berger and Berger, *War over the Family*, 3, 65–66, 102, 109.

9. Tillich, *The Courage to Be*, 26–27.

10. Goldscheider and Waite, *New Families, No Families*, 202.

11. Chopp, "Feminist Theology," 191.

12. Snitow, "Feminism and Motherhood," 35–38. Feminist writing in all fields, including theology, cannot be exactly aligned with Snitow's time line. On the other hand, Snitow demonstrates that within the ebb and flow of feminist writing on motherhood there is a gradual development toward inclusiveness of an ever-widening set of perspectives.

13. Dally, *Inventing Motherhood*, 177–78.

14. Firestone, *Dialectic of Sex*, 188–89.

15. Leach, *Who Cares?*, 40.

16. Dally, *Inventing Motherhood*, 177.

17. Miller-McLemore, *Also a Mother*, 89.

18. "Introduction: Womanspirit Rising," in Christ and Plaskow, *Womanspirit Rising*, 3–9.

19. Christ, "Margaret Atwood," 316–20.

20. Snitow, "Feminism and Motherhood," 34.

21. Rich, *Of Woman Born*, 109, 116.

22. Scarr, *Mother Care, Other Care*, 101.

23. Lamb et al., "Varying Degrees of Paternal Involvement in Infant Care," 117–38; Russell, "Shared-Caregiving Families," 139–71; Radin, "Primary Caregiving and Role-Sharing Fathers," 173–204; and Sagi, "Antecedents and Consequences of Various Degrees of Paternal Involvement in Child Rearing," 139–71.

24. Hochschild, *The Second Shift*.

25. Goldscheider and Waite, *New Families, No Families*, 201.

26. Snitow, "Feminism and Motherhood," 42.

27. Goldscheider and Waite (*New Families, No Families*, 201) note that this has devastating effects on all family members. It especially affects boys who grow up without contact with real men and are left to try to pattern their own lives on those of stereotypes fostered by the media. This does not augur well for the future families of these boys.

28. Cardozo, *Sequencing*, xi.

29. Snitow, "Feminism and Motherhood," 44.

30. Okin, *Justice, Gender, and the Family*, 176.

31. Miller-McLemore, *Also a Mother*, 55–57.

32. Goldscheider and Waite, *New Families, No Families*, xiii.

33. Miller-McLemore, *Also a Mother*, 74; also see Rothman, *Recreating Motherhood*, 20, and part 1 in general.

34. Rothman, *Recreating Motherhood*, 88–89.

35. "A Conversation with Valerie Saiving," 100.

36. Dally, *Inventing Motherhood*, 189–90, 197.

37. Miller-McLemore, *Also a Mother*, 170. See also Chodorow and Cantratto, *Reproduction of Mothering*; Dinnerstein, *The Mermaid and the Minotaur*.

38. It is interesting to note that in some other cultures the "triad" is considered the mother, child, and household, with the father being sometimes excluded from the last as far as infant care is concerned. See Winikoff, Castle, and Hight-Laukaron, *Feeding Infants in Four Societies*.

39. Jackson, *Mother Zone*, 75–83.

40. Fiorenza, *In Memory of Her*, 350.

41. Okin, *Justice, Gender, and the Family*, 116.

42. Scarr, *Mother Care, Other Care*, 206–7.

43. Miller-McLemore, *Also a Mother*, 153.

44. Ibid., 157.

45. Ibid., 157–84.

46. Charles Leroux and Cindy Schreuder, *Chicago Tribune* staff writers, suggest that there are two possible reasons why mother-infant relationships have been given more attention than father-child relationships: "One reason is that the parent who gave birth long has been thought to have the stronger ties to the newborn. Another is more mundane: Researchers prefer not to work nights and weekends when dads are more likely to be home." See Leroux and Schreuder, "Handle with Care," *Chicago Tribune*, October 30, 1994, sec. 1, 9.

CHAPTER 5

1. La Leche League International, *Womanly Art of Breastfeeding*, 3d ed., 7, 133.

2. Riordan and Auerbach, *Breastfeeding and Human Lactation*, 241.

3. La Leche League International, *Womanly Art of Breastfeeding*, 3d ed., 96.

4. Plummer, review of *Oneness and Separateness*, 11.

5. Kaplan, *Oneness and Separateness*, 15.

6. Ibid., 19.

7. Stanton, review of *Who Cares for the Baby?*, 36.

8. Kaplan, *Oneness and Separateness*, 37–38.

9. La Leche League International, *Womanly Art of Breastfeeding*, 3d ed., 95.

10. Ibid.

11. Abruzzi, "What Nursing Has Meant to Me," 5.

12. Kaplan, *Oneness and Separateness*, 78–79.

13. Wilson, "Musings," 5.

14. Friesen, "The Welcoming of Jonathan," 17–18.

15. Kaplan, *Oneness and Separateness*, 85–88.

16. Ibid., 118–19.

17. Mary Ann Cahill, "Mother-Baby Separation," 17.

18. Good and Phillips, "How Leaders Help Mothers," 25–26.

19. La Leche League International, *Womanly Art of Breastfeeding*, 2d ed., 109.

20. Hahn, "Mothering," 27.

21. Lynne Emerson, quoted in La Leche League International, *Womanly Art of Breastfeeding*, 3d ed., 118.

22. La Leche League International, *Womanly Art of Breastfeeding*, 3d ed., 67.

23. Mary White interview. This perspective is understandable when one considers that White is the mother of twelve. Her first grandchild was born before her youngest daughter. Also, this grandson was born in White's home. In addition, White has been a vocal, active member of the La Leche League's board since its inception.

24. Burton, Dittmer, and Loveless, *What's a Smart Woman Like You Doing at Home?*, 114.

25. Rich, *Of Woman Born*, 192.

26. Mary Ann Cahill, *The Heart Has Its Own Reasons*, 113.

27. Lowman, *Of Cradles and Careers*, 4–5, 112, 149–51.

28. Herbert Ratner, introduction to Founding Mothers, *La Leche League Dialogue*, 5.

29. La Leche League International, *Womanly Art of Breastfeeding*, 3d ed., 8.

30. World Health Organization, 1979 statement on breast feeding, quoted in La Leche League International, *Womanly Art of Breastfeeding*, 3d ed., 8.

31. Harris, "Physicians and Leader," n.p.

32. La Leche League International, "Helping Mothers and Babies Everywhere," 1.

33. "La Leche League Goes to Prison," 55–56.

34. La Leche League International, *Womanly Art of Breastfeeding*, 3d ed., 145.

35. Gilligan, *In a Different Voice*, 1, 8, 16–19.

36. Constantino, "The Essence of La Leche League," 67–68.

37. Ladas, "How to Help Mothers Breastfeed," 702–4.

38. Members of the team were Kathleen Astin-Knaff, Roger D. Irle, Ruth Shonie Cavan, Linda Dammers, and Claronette M. Booker.

39. Meara lists these perspectives as (1) breast feeding soon after delivery, (2) breast feeding on demand at the hospital, (3) rooming-in at the hospital, (4) breast feeding on demand at home, (5) introducing first solids at 4–6 months, (6) gradual and cooperative weaning, and (7) nursing longer than nine months.

40. Meara, "Key to Successful Breast-Feeding," 20–26.

41. Miller-McLemore, *Also a Mother*, 30.

CHAPTER 6

1. "Praxis" as I use it here adheres closely to Thomas Groome's definition of praxis as "the consciousness and agency that arise from and are expressed in any and every aspect of people's 'being' as agent-subjects-in-relationship, whether realized in actions that are personal, interpersonal, sociopolitical, or cosmic." See Groome, *Sharing Faith*, 136.

2. "Texts" here means not only the League's writings but also its practices.

3. Tracy, *Analogical Imagination*, 70.

4. Schuck, "Content and Coherence of Roman Catholic Encyclical Social Teaching," 114, 406–7.

5. Campion, "The Church Today," 183.

6. *Child and Family Digest* is owned, edited, and published quarterly by the National Commission on Human Life, Reproduction and Rhythm. At the time of La Leche League's founding, its editor was Dr. Herbert Ratner.

7. This concept has had and continues to have many interpretations within the American context. I investigate the one that most directly affected La Leche League theory because it was the most prevalent pastoral interpretation at midcentury.

8. Lisa Sowle Cahill, *Between the Sexes*, 110.

9. Leo XIII, *Libertas*, 8 (2:171). Unless otherwise noted, all citations referring to the papal encyclicals in this and the following chapters are taken from Carlen, *Papal Encyclicals*. The numbers appearing after encyclical titles refer to the paragraph numbers used in the Carlen translations. They are followed by the volume and page numbers.

10. Pius XI, *Non Abbiamo Bisogno*, 27 (3:451).

11. Davis, *Moral and Pastoral Theology*, 126–27.

12. Schuck names this period as 1959 to the present and notes that it is so called because "current encyclical commentators note significant departures from Leonine period encyclical teaching beginning in the letters of John XXIII."

13. John XXIII, *Ad Petri Cathedram*, 51 (5:10).

14. Pius XII, *Sertum Laetitiae*, 22 (3:31).

15. Greeley, *The Catholic Myth*, 96–100. This was the year of the publication of *Humanae Vitae*, but as Greeley points out, this encyclical alone cannot explain the ensuing confusion about the birth control issue. The Second Vatican Council had earlier declared, "Human beings should be judiciously informed of scientific advances in the exploration of methods by which spouses can be helped in arranging the number of their children" (*Constitution of the Church in the Modern World*, in Abbott, *Documents of Vatican II*, 302). The church seemed to contradict itself. However, La Leche League's founders were traditional Catholics, and the earlier attitude parallels their own beliefs about the importance of children within families. They do not take a stand on birth control per se, but, as will be described in the next chapter, they do stress the delayed fertility aspects of breast feeding.

16. Dohen, *Women in Wonderland*, 104, 106–7.

17. Ibid., 21.

18. Aquinas, *Summa Theologiae* (1, Q. 92, a, 1). A similar understanding of the nature of women is found in Augustine's *The Literal Meaning of Genesis* (*De Genesi ad literam*), ix, 3.

19. Leo XIII, *Rerum Novarum*, 36, 42, 43 (2:250–53).

20. Dohen, *Women in Wonderland*, 31–46.

21. Zappone, "Woman's Special Nature," 87–90.

22. Kenneally, *History of American Catholic Women*, 178–88.

23. Leo XIII, *Arcanum*, 11 (2:32).

24. Kenneally, *History of American Catholic Women*, 191.

25. Dohen, *Women in Wonderland*, 89.

26. Pius XI, *Casti Connubii*, 24 (3:395).

27. Pope, "Order of Love," 257.

28. Ibid., 99.

29. Hardon, *Catholic Catechism*, 194–96.

30. Browning, *Fundamental Practical Theology*, 161.

31. Janssens, "Norms and Priorities in a Love Ethic," 212-15.

32. Vatican II and Paul VI, *Lumen Gentium* (October 20, 1962), in Abbott, *Documents of Vatican II*, 88.

33. Pius IX, *Qui Pluribus*, 36 (1:284).

34. Pius XII, *Mystici Corporis Christi*, 110 (4:60).

35. John XXIII, *Grata Recordatio*, 10 (5:40).

36. Paul VI and Vatican II, *Lumen Gentium*, 55, in Flannery, *Conciliar and Post Conciliar Documents*, 415-19.

37. Abbott, *Documents of Vatican II*, 85 n. 256.

38. Pius IX, *Ubi Primum*, 5 (1:292).

39. Paul VI and Vatican II, *Lumen Gentium*, 65, in Flannery, *Conciliar and Post Conciliar Documents*, 397-99, 420.

40. Kenneally, *History of American Catholic Women*, 161, 188.

41. Kassel, "Mary and the Human Psyche," 77.

42. Redmont, *Generous Lives*, 104.

43. Three notable popular Catholic successes were Bishop Fulton Sheen's television program, Franz Werfel's *Song of Bernadette*, and Thomas Merton's book, *The Seven Story Mountain*. The very revival of anti-Catholic sentiment, epitomized by Paul Blanshard's *American Freedom and Catholic Power*, testified to the nation's new awareness of the Catholic community. For a discussion of these works, see Brown, *Grail Movement in American Catholicism*.

44. Brown, *Grail Movement in American Catholicism*. Consistency of doctrine is apparent here, as the bishops' statement alludes to the stance taken by Pius XI in *Casti Connubii* in 1931.

45. Dohen, *Women in Wonderland*, 107.

46. This organization would later change its name to the Christian Family Movement, but at the time of the founders' initial involvement, it was still called the Catholic Family Movement.

47. Kenneally, *History of American Catholic Women*, 188; Dolan, *American Catholic Experience*, 395.

CHAPTER 7

1. Although these convictions were most apparent in the League's earliest writings, they span the movement and continue to appear in League literature. Here I focus on the early literature but have included selections from more recent writings to indicate the League's consistent adherence to these notions.

2. Founding Mothers, *La Leche League Dialogue*, 23.

3. La Leche League International, *Womanly Art of Breastfeeding*, 2d ed., 2.

4. Ibid., 1st ed., 8.

5. Ibid., 2d ed., 11.

6. Founding Mothers, *La Leche League Dialogue*, 54.

7. Ibid., 12.

8. Mary Ann Cahill interview.

9. La Leche League International, *Womanly Art of Breastfeeding*, 1st ed., 5.

10. Rookey, "All-Natural Ice Milk," 149.

11. La Leche League International, *Womanly Art of Breastfeeding*, 1st ed., 22.

12. Romano, "Oxytocin," 78-79.

13. La Leche League International, *Womanly Art of Breastfeeding*, 3d ed., 95.

14. Eskuchen, "Parenting Styles," 42.

15. Crase, "Making Your Wishes Come True," 82.

16. La Leche League International, *Womanly Art of Breastfeeding*, 1st ed., 19–29.

17. Gotsch, "Daddies Are for Fun," 115.

18. Cardozo, *Sequencing*, 79–80.

19. Dave Stewart, title not given, *La Leche League News* (n.d.), quoted in La Leche League International, *Womanly Art of Breastfeeding*, 3d ed., 158. While this manual contains many excellent quotes, references are scanty and there are no footnotes. Also early editions of the *La Leche League News* were not originally minutely indexed.

20. Mayer, "Loving Partner," 177.

21. Bobman, "Romantic Ride," 20.

22. La Leche League International, *Womanly Art of Breastfeeding*, 3d ed., 18.

23. These women's narratives are included in the second edition of the manual. All are referred to by first names only.

24. Donna Bryant, "A Change of Plans," in Mary Ann Cahill, *The Heart Has Its Own Reasons*, 335–37.

25. La Leche League International, *Womanly Art of Breastfeeding*, 2d ed., 4.

26. Varencov, "Nursing Madonna."

27. Taylor, "Duty of Nursing Children," 27.

28. The beliefs and feelings of the founding mothers about Mary were gathered by the author in a series of interviews conducted in March 1993.

29. Scheff, "What Is Development?," 146.

30. Ibid.

31. White, "Full Circle," 110.

32. Founding Mothers, *La Leche League Dialogue*, 46–49.

33. The beliefs and feelings of the founding mothers about the CFM were gathered by the author in a series of interviews conducted in March 1993.

34. Unidentified founding mother, in Founding Mothers, *La Leche League Dialogue*, 18.

35. Gotsch, "Can Breastfeeding Become the Cultural Norm?," 163–68.

36. Lewis, "Managerial Nursing," 40.

37. White, "Full Circle," 110.

38. Everman, "Making a Choice," 177–78.

39. The beliefs and feelings of the founding mothers about the League's Catholic origins and regarding its stance on abortion were gathered by the author in a series of interviews conducted in March 1993.

CHAPTER 8

1. Groome, *Sharing Faith*, 136.

2. Eliade, *The Sacred and the Profane*, 12.

3. Herbert Ratner, introduction to La Leche League International, *Womanly Art of Breastfeeding*, 3d ed., x.

4. Ibid., xi.

5. Mahler, Pine, and Bergman, *Psychological Birth of the Human Infant*, 225–30.

6. Mayo, "Breast or Bottle?," 38–40.

7. In his *Pensées*, Pascal first emphasized that "if we offend the principles of reason, our religion will be absurd and ridiculous." He goes on to say, however, "The heart has its reasons which reason does not know. We feel it in a thousand things. I say the heart naturally loves the Universal Being. . . . God is felt by the heart, not by reason" (44–45).

8. John XXIII, *Pacem in Terris*, 153, 151 (5:124); *Mater et Magistra*, 198 (5:81).

9. Andrews, "Controlling Motherhood," 87.

10. La Leche League International, *Womanly Art of Breastfeeding*, 3d ed., 338.

11. Ibid., xxvii, 100, 110, 145, 188. Brewster (*You Can Breastfeed Your Baby*) does note that there are exceptions to this rule, such as infants with malformation of the nose, mouth, or digestive tract. It is possible to see that these babies receive their mothers' milk; however, she writes, the "tremendous strain and . . . pressure" on the family can make bottle feeding the "less traumatic" choice in these circumstances (169). Interestingly, Brewster quotes Reinhold Niebuhr's "Serenity Prayer" when she addresses the question of "what qualifies as an upsetting situation . . . to a nursing mother" (455).

12. Borresen, "Mary in Catholic Theology," 53.

13. Marian Tompson interview.

14. Whelan, *Living Strings*, 135.

15. Greeley, *The Mary Myth*, 13. South American Christianity also offers a powerful example. The Spanish conquest and religious conversion of native South Americans had resulted in a political-economic, sexual, sociopsychological, and religious oppression. Yet, within this "context of death and despair a divine irruption takes place far away from the centers of power of the State or of established religion." This was the apparition of the "Indian Queen of Heaven" to Juan Diego, a poor Nahuath Indian. "Today the oppressed of Latin America continue to find security and hope through devotions to Our Lady of Guadalupe." See Elizondo, "Mary and the Poor," 60–61.

16. Whelan, *Living Strings*, 135.

17. Borresen, "Mary in Catholic Theology," 49–50.

18. Halkes, "Mary and Women," 69.

19. Mananzan, "Education to Femininity or Feminism?," 31.

20. Halkes, "Mary and Women," 68.

21. La Leche League International, *Womanly Art of Breastfeeding*, 2d ed., 141.

22. Browning, *Religious Thought and the Modern Psychologies*, 126.

23. Gudorf, *Liberation Themes*, 255.

24. Kenneally, *History of American Catholic Women*, 161, 189.

25. Okin, *Justice, Gender, and the Family*, 170–71.

26. Brewster, *You Can Breastfeed Your Baby*, 27.

27. Newman, "Mutual Respect in the Health Care Community." Tapes of Newman's presentation are available from La Leche League International, 1400 N. Meacham Road, Schaumburg, IL 60173-4840.

28. Froehlich, "Nurturing the World through Nurturing Our Families." Tapes of Froehlich's presentation are available from La Leche League International, 1400 N. Meacham Road, Schaumburg, IL 60173-4840.

29. Thevenin, "Mothering and Fathering." Tapes of Thevenin's presentation are available from La Leche League International, 1400 N. Meacham Road, Schaumburg, IL 60173-4840.

30. Fazal, "The Rebirth of Breastfeeding Worldwide." Tapes of Fazal's presentation are available from La Leche League International, 1400 N. Meacham Road, Schaumburg, IL 60173-4840.

31. Hunter, *In the Company of Women*.

32. Pope, "Order of Love," 263.

33. Mary Ann Cahill, *The Heart Has Its Own Reasons*, 28.

34. Pope, "Order of Love," 267.

35. Adago, "Vigil of Hope," 39.

36. Pope, "Order of Love," 274.

37. Black, "The Medicalization of Breastfeeding and Other Intrusions into Motherhood." Tapes of Black's presentation are available from La Leche League International, 1400 N. Meacham Road, Schaumburg, IL 60173-4840.

38. Ibid.

CHAPTER 9

1. Andrews, "Controlling Motherhood," 84–85, 95.

2. Black, "The Medicalization of Breastfeeding and Other Intrusions into Motherhood." Tapes of Black's presentation are available from La Leche League International.

3. Newman, "Mutual Respect in the Health Care Community." (Newman cites *Pediatrics* 88 [1991]: 1055 and Judson, *Artificial Feeding*.) Tapes of Newman's presentation are available from La Leche League International.

4. Ibid. (Newman cites Lowenburn, *Infant Feeding*, and refers to the entire October 1993 issue of *Pediatric Nursing* as a good reference.)

5. Freed, "Time to Teach What We Preach," 243–44. Freed cites Applebaum, "Obstetrician's Approach," 98–116.

6. Pogash, "War between Women," C4.

7. Sayers, *Biological Politics*, 3–4.

8. Becker, "Maternal Feelings," 142–67.

9. Lopez et al., "Establishment of Mother-to-Mother Support." Tapes of Lopez et al.'s presentation are available from La Leche League International, 1400 N. Meacham Road, Schaumburg, IL 60173-4840. This group continued their discussion at the Fifteenth International Conference in Washington, D.C., in July 1997. These tapes are not yet available.

10. NETWORK, *Shaping a New World*, 2.

11. Schuck, "Content and Coherence of Roman Catholic Encyclical Social Teaching," 371–73.

12. Coleman, *One Hundred Years of Catholic Social Thought*, 160.

13. Lowman, *Of Cradles and Careers*, 182.

14. Hellwig, *Understanding Catholicism*, 185.

15. Locklin, "Passionate Advocacy," 181.

16. John Paul II, *Laborum Exercens*, 6 (5:304).

17. Kuttner, "Worker Rights and Responsibilities," 234–39.

18. John Paul II, *Laborum Exercens*, 5:299.

19. Mary Ann Cahill, *The Heart Has Its Own Reasons*, 43, 48, 52, 55.

20. Miller, "Centennial Encyclical," 10.

21. Palmer, *Politics of Breastfeeding*, 2, 6.

22. Rivers, "New School of Thought," 5, 1.

23. Navin, "Remarkable Leader," 84.

24. Townsend, "Breastfeeding Gains Popularity in Honduras," 15–17.

25. Fazal, "The Rebirth of Breastfeeding Worldwide."

26. Herbert Ratner, introduction to La Leche League International, *Womanly Art of Breastfeeding*, 3d ed., xii.

bibliography

· ·

BOOKS

Abbott, Walter M., gen. ed. Joseph Gallagher, trans. ed. *The Documents of Vatican II*. New York: Guild Press, 1966.

Albanese, Catherine L. *Nature Religion in America: From the Algonkian Indians to the New Age*. Chicago: University of Chicago Press, 1990.

Apple, Rima D. *Mothers and Medicine: A Social History of Infant Feeding, 1890–1950*. Madison: University of Wisconsin Press, 1987.

Aquinas, Thomas. *Summa Theologiae*. Vol. 13. Edited and translated by Edmund Hill. New York: McGraw-Hill, 1963.

Arcana, Judith. *Our Mothers' Daughters*. Berkeley, Calif.: Shameless Hussy Press, 1979.

Augustine. *The Literal Meaning of Genesis*. Vol. 2. Edited and translated by John Hammond Taylor. New York: Newman Press, 1982.

Badinter, Elizabeth. *Mother Love: Myth and Reality*. New York: Macmillan, 1980.

Barrett, Michele, and Mary McIntosh. *The Anti-Social Family*. London: Verso, 1982.

Berger, Brigitte, and Peter L. Berger. *The War over the Family*. Garden City, N.Y.: Anchor Books, 1983.

Bernerd, Jessie. *The Future of Motherhood*. New York: Dial Press, 1974.

Boston Women's Health Course Collective. *Our Bodies, Ourselves*. Boston: New England Free Press, 1971.

Brewster, Dorothy P. *You Can Breastfeed Your Baby — Even in Special Circumstances*. Foreword by Derrick B. Jelliffe. Emmaus, Pa.: Rodale Press, 1979.

Brown, Alden V. *The Grail Movement in American Catholicism, 1940–1975*. Notre Dame, Ind.: University of Notre Dame Press, 1989.

Browning, Don S. *A Fundamental Practical Theology: Descriptive and Strategic Proposals*. Minneapolis: Fortress Press, 1991.

———. *Religious Thought and the Modern Psychologies*. Philadelphia: Fortress Press, 1987.

Burton, Linda, Janet Dittmer, and Cheri Loveless. *What's a Smart Woman Like You Doing at Home?* Washington, D.C.: Acropolis Books, 1986.

Cahill, Lisa Sowle. *Between the Sexes: Foundations for a Christian Ethics of Sexuality.* Philadelphia: Fortress Press, 1985.

——. *Sex, Gender, and Christian Ethics.* New York: Cambridge University Press, 1996.

Cahill, Mary Ann. *The Heart Has Its Own Reasons: Mothering Wisdom for the 1980s.* Franklin Park, Ill.: La Leche League International, 1983.

Cardozo, Arlene. *Sequencing.* New York: Collier, 1986.

Carr, Anne E. *Transforming Grace: Christian Tradition and Women's Experience.* San Francisco: Harper and Row, 1988.

Chesler, Phyllis. *With Child: A Diary of Motherhood.* New York: Thomas Y. Crowell, 1979.

Chodorow, Nancy, and Susan Cantratto. *The Reproduction of Mothering: Psychoanalysis and the Sociology of Gender.* Berkeley: University of California Press, 1978.

Christ, Carol, and Judith Plaskow, eds. *Womanspirit Rising.* San Francisco: Harper and Row, 1979.

Coleman, John A., ed. *One Hundred Years of Catholic Social Thought.* Maryknoll, N.Y.: Orbis, 1990.

Cott, Nancy. *The Bonds of Womanhood.* New Haven, Conn.: Yale University Press, 1977.

Curran, Charles. *Contemporary Problems in Moral Theology.* Notre Dame, Ind.: Fides, 1970.

Dally, Ann. *Inventing Motherhood.* New York: Schocken, 1983.

Davis, Henry. *Moral and Pastoral Theology.* Vol. 1. New York: Sheed and Ward, 1959.

Degler, Carl. *At Odds: Women and the Family in America from the Revolution to the Present.* New York: Oxford University Press, 1980.

Department of Religious Studies, DePaul University. *Religious Worlds: Primary Readings in Comparative Perspective.* Edited by John Dominic Crossan. Chicago: De Paul University Press, 1991.

Dinnerstein, Dorothy. *The Mermaid and the Minotaur.* New York: Harper and Row, 1976.

Dohen, Dorothy. *Women in Wonderland.* New York: Sheed and Ward, 1960.

Dolan, Jay P. *The American Catholic Experience.* Garden City, N.Y.: Doubleday, 1985.

Durkin, Mary. *The Suburban Woman: Her Changing Role in the Church.* New York: Seabury Press, 1974.

Eliade, Mircea. *The Sacred and the Profane.* Translated by Willard R. Trask. New York: Harcourt Brace Jovanovich, 1959.

Ellul, Jacques. *The Technological Society.* New York: Vintage, 1964.

Fiorenza, Elisabeth Schussler. *In Memory of Her: A Feminist Theological Reconstruction of Christian Origins.* New York: Crossroads, 1985.

Firestone, Shulamith. *The Dialectic of Sex.* London: Paladin, 1972.

Flannery, Austin, ed. *The Conciliar and Post Conciliar Documents.* Rev. ed. Collegeville, Ind.: Liturgical Press, 1992.

Ford, John C., and Gerald Kelly. *Contemporary Moral Theology: Marriage Questions.* Westminster, Md.: Newman, 1963.

Founding Mothers. *A La Leche League Dialogue: An Historic Document.* Introduction by Herbert Ratner. Oak Park, Ill.: Child and Family, 1981.

Frank, Jerome. *Persuasion and Healing: A Comparative Study of Psychotherapy*. New York: Schocken, 1974.

Friedan, Betty. *The Feminine Mystique*. New York: W. W. Norton, 1963.

Geertz, Clifford. *The Interpretation of Cultures*. New York: Basic Books, 1973.

Gerber Products. *The Incredible, Insatiable Sucking Desire*. Fremont, Mich.: Gerber Products, 1994.

Gerson, Kathleen. *Hard Choices: How Women Decide about Work, Career, and Motherhood*. Berkeley: University of California Press, 1985.

Gilligan, Carol. *In a Different Voice: Psychological Theory and Women's Development*. Cambridge, Mass.: Harvard University Press, 1982.

Goldscheider, Frances, and Linda Waite. *New Families, No Families*. Berkeley: University of California Press, 1991.

Greeley, Andrew. *The Catholic Myth*. New York: Charles Scribner's Sons, 1990.

———. *The Mary Myth: On the Femininity of God*. New York: Seabury Press, 1977.

Green, Christopher. *Dr. Green's Baby Book*. New York: Fawcett Columbine, 1988.

Groome, Thomas. *Sharing Faith*. San Francisco: Harper San Francisco, 1991.

Gudorf, Christine. *Liberation Themes*. Washington, D.C.: University Press of America, 1981.

Habermas, Jürgen. *The Theory of Communicative Action*. Vol. 1. Translated by Thomas McCarthy. Boston: Beacon Press, 1984.

Hammer, Signe. *Daughters and Mothers, Mothers and Daughters*. New York: Quadrangle, 1975.

Hardon, John A. *The Catholic Catechism: A Contemporary Catechism of the Teachings of the Catholic Church*. New York: Doubleday, 1981.

Hayes, Royal Storrs. *Infant and Child Feeding*. New York and London: D. Appleton, 1928.

Hellwig, Monica. *Understanding Catholicism*. New York: Paulist Press, 1981.

Hennesey, James. *American Catholics: A History of the Roman Catholic Community in America*. New York: Oxford University Press, 1981.

Hewlett, Sylvia Ann. *A Lesser Life: The Myth of Women's Liberation in America*. New York: William Morrow, 1986.

Hochschild, Arlie. *The Second Shift*. New York: Avon, 1989.

Hoffner, Elaine. *Mothering: The Emotional Experience of Motherhood after Freud and Feminism*. New York: Doubleday, 1978.

Howard, Jane. *Families*. New York: Simon and Schuster, 1978.

Hunter, Brenda M. *In the Company of Women*. Sisters, Oreg.: Questar, 1994.

Jackson, Marni. *The Mother Zone: Love, Sex, and Laundry in the Modern Family*. New York: Henry Holt, 1992.

James, William. *The Varieties of Religious Experience*. New York: Doubleday, 1978.

Jelliffe, D. B., and E. F. Jelliffe. *Human Milk in the Modern World*. Oxford: Oxford University Press, 1977.

Judson, Charles Francis. *The Artificial Feeding of Infants*. Philadelphia: Lippincott, 1902.

Kahel, Judy, and Lorrie Dyal, eds. *Leader's Handbook*. Franklin Park, Ill.: La Leche League International, 1977.

Kaplan, Louise. *Oneness and Separateness: From Infant to Individual*. Foreword by Margaret S. Mahler. New York: Simon and Schuster, 1978.

Kenneally, James J. *The History of American Catholic Women*. New York: Crossroad Press, 1990.

Kippley, Sheila. *Breast Feeding and Natural Child Spacing*. New York: Harper and Row, 1974.

Klaus, M. H. *Maternal-Infant Bonding*. St. Louis: Mosby, 1976.

Kung, Hans, and Jürgen Moltmann, eds. *Mary in the Churches*. Concilium, vol. 168. New York: Seabury Press, 1983.

La Leche League International. *The Womanly Art of Breastfeeding*. 1st ed. Franklin Park, Ill.: La Leche League International, 1956.

——. *The Womanly Art of Breastfeeding*. 2d ed. Foreword by Herbert Ratner. Franklin Park, Ill.: La Leche League International, 1958.

——. *The Womanly Art of Breastfeeding*. 3d ed. Introduction by Herbert Ratner. Foreword by Niles Newton. Franklin Park, Ill.: La Leche League International, 1981.

Lancaster, Jane B., Jeanne Altmann, Alice S. Rossi, and Lonnie R. Sherrod, eds. *Parenting across the Life Span: Biosocial Dimension*. New York: Aldine de Gruyter, 1990.

Lasch, Christopher. *Haven in a Heartless World: The Family Besieged*. New York: Basic Books, 1977.

Laslett, Peter, ed. *Household and Family in Past Time*. Cambridge: Cambridge University Press, 1972.

Leach, Penelope. *Who Cares? A New Deal for Mothers and Their Small Children*. London: Penguin, 1979.

Lowenburn, Harry. *Infant Feeding and Allied Topics*. Philadelphia: F. A. David, 1916.

Lowman, Kaye. *The LLLove Story*. Franklin Park, Ill.: La Leche League International, 1977.

——. *Of Cradles and Careers: A Guide to Reshaping Your Job to Include a Baby in Your Life*. Franklin Park, Ill.: La Leche League International, 1984.

McCann, Dennis, and Charles Strain. *Polity and Praxis: A Program for American Practical Theology*. Minneapolis: Winston Press, 1985.

Mackin, Theodore. *Marriage in the Catholic Church*. 3 vols. Mahwah, N.J.: Paulist Press. Vol. 1, *What Is Marriage?* (1982); vol. 2, *Divorce and Remarriage* (1984); vol. 3, *The Marital Sacrament* (1989).

Mahler, Margaret S., Fred Pine, and Anni Bergman. *The Psychological Birth of the Human Infant*. New York: Basic Books, 1975.

Markel, Howard, and Frank A. Oski. *The H. L. Mencken Baby Book*. Philadelphia: Hanley and Belfus, 1990.

May, Charles D., ed. *Better Homes and Gardens Baby Book: A Handbook for Parents*. 5th rev. ed. Des Moines, Iowa: Meredith, 1956.

Miller-McLemore, Bonnie. *Also a Mother*. Nashville: Abingdon Press, 1994.

Niebuhr, Reinhold. *The Nature and Destiny of Man*. Vol. 2. New York: Charles Scribner's Sons, 1941.

NETWORK, a National Catholic Social Justice Lobby. *Shaping a New World*. Washington, D.C.: NETWORK, 1991.

Newton, Niles. *The Family Book of Child Care*. New York: Harper and Row, 1957.

Nygren, Anders. *Agape and Eros*. Philadelphia: Westminster Press, 1953.

O'Connell, Timothy E. *Principles for a Catholic Morality*. San Francisco: Harper and Row, 1976.

Okin, Susan Moller. *Justice, Gender, and the Family*. New York: Basic Books, 1989.

Oppenheimer, Valerie. *Work and the Family*. New York: Academic Press, 1982.

Packard, Veenal S. *Human Milk and Infant Formula*. New York: Academic Press, 1982.

Palmer, Gabrielle. *The Politics of Breastfeeding*. London: Pandora Press, 1988.

Pascal, Blaise. *Pensées*. In *Great Books of the Western World*, vol. 30. Edited by Clifton Fadiman and Philip W. Goetz, translated by W. C. Trotter. Chicago: Encyclopedia Brittanica, 1990.

Popkin, Barry, Tamar Lasky, Judith Litvin, Deborah Spicer, and Monica Yamaoto. *The Infant-Feeding Triad: Infant, Mother, and Household*. New York: Gordon and Breach Science, 1986.

Pryor, Karen. *Nursing Your Baby*. New York: Harper and Row, 1963.

Raphael, Daphne. *The Tender Gift: Breastfeeding*. New York: Schocken, 1976.

Redmont, Jane. *Generous Lives*. Liguori, Mo.: Triumph Books, 1992.

Rich, Adrienne. *Of Woman Born: Motherhood as Experience and Institution*. New York: W. W. Norton, 1976.

Riordan, Jan, and Kathleen G. Auerbach. *Breastfeeding and Human Lactation*. Boston: Jones and Bartlett, 1993.

Rothman, Barbara Katz. *Recreating Motherhood: Ideology and Technology in a Patriarchal Society*. New York: W. W. Norton, 1989.

Ruether, Rosemary R. *Mary: The Feminine Face of the Church*. Philadelphia: Westminster Press, 1972.

Saxton, Stanley, Patricia Voydanoff, and Angela A. Zukowski, eds. *The Changing Family*. Chicago: Loyola University Press, 1982.

Sayers, Janet. *Biological Politics*. London: Tavistock, 1982.

Scarr, Sandra. *Mother Care, Other Care*. New York: Basic Books, 1984.

Schillebeeckx, E. *Marriage: Human Reality and Saving Mystery*. New York: Sheed and Ward, 1965.

Smith, Lendon H. *The Encyclopedia of Baby and Child Care*. Englewood Cliffs, N.J.: Prentice-Hall, 1972.

Spock, Benjamin. *The Common Sense Book of Baby and Child Care*. New York: Duell, Sloan, and Pearce, 1946.

Tentler, Leslie. *Wage-Earning Women*. New York: Oxford University Press, 1979.

Terman, Lewis Madison, and Catherine Miles. *Sex and Personality Studies in Masculinity and Femininity*. New York: McGraw-Hill, 1936.

Tillich, Paul. *The Courage to Be*. New Haven, Conn.: Yale University Press, 1952.

———. *Systematic Theology*. Vol. 1. Chicago: University of Chicago Press, 1951.

Tracy, David. *The Analogical Imagination*. New York: Crossroad Publishing, 1987.

———. *Blessed Rage for Order*. Minneapolis: Winston-Seabury Press, 1975.

Whelan, Michael. *Living Strings*. Newtown, NSW, Australia: E. J. Dwyer, 1994.

Winikoff, Beverly, Mary Ann Castle, and Virginia Hight-Laukaron, eds. *Feeding Infants in Four Societies: Causes and Consequences of Mothers' Choices*. New York: Greenwood Press, 1988.

World Health Organization. *Contemporary Patterns in Breast-Feeding: Report on the WHO Collaborative Study on Breast-Feeding*. Geneva: World Health Organization, 1981.

PAPAL ENCYCLICALS

Carlen, Claudia, ed. *The Papal Encyclicals: 1740–1978*. Raleigh, N.C.: McGrath Publishing, 1981. (This five-volume work is the source for the papal encyclicals cited in this work.)

Pius VIII. *Traditi Humilitati.* May 24, 1829, 1:221–24.

Pius IX. *Qui Pluribus.* November 9, 1846, 1:278–84.

———. *Ubi Primum.* February 2, 1849, 1:291–93.

———. *Nostis et Nobiscum.* December 8, 1849, 1:295–303.

Leo XIII. *Arcanum.* February 10, 1880, 2:29–40.

———. *Libertas.* June 20, 1888, 2:169–81.

———. *Rerum Novarum.* January 6, 1895, 2:241–61.

Pius XI. *Ubi Arcano Dei Consilio.* December 23, 1922, 3:225–39.

———. *Rappresentanti in Terra.* December 31, 1929, 3:353–71.

———. *Casti Connubii.* December 31, 1930, 3:391–414.

———. *Quadragesimo Anno.* May 15, 1931, 3:415–43.

———. *Non Abbiamo Bisogno.* June 29, 1931, 3:445–58.

Pius XII. *Summi Pontificatus.* October 20, 1939, 4:5–22.

———. *Sertum Laetitiae.* November 1, 1939, 3:23–30.

———. *Mystici Corporis Christi.* June 29, 1943, 4:37–63.

John XXIII. *Ad Petri Cathedram.* June 29, 1959, 5:5–20.

———. *Grata Recordatio.* September 26, 1959, 5:39–41.

———. *Mater et Magistra.* May 15, 1961, 5:59–90.

———. *Pacem in Terris.* April 11, 1963, 5:107–29.

Paul VI. *Ecclesiam Suam.* August 6, 1964, 5:135–60.

———. *Populorium Progressio.* March 26, 1967, 5:83–201.

———. *Sacerdotalis Caelibatus.* June 24, 1967, 5:203–21.

———. *Humanae Vitae.* July 25, 1968, 5:223–36.

John Paul II. *Redemptor Hominis.* March 4, 1979, 5:245–73.

———. *Dives in Misericordii.* November 30, 1980, 5:276–98.

———. *Laborum Exercens.* September 14, 1981, 5:299–326.

JOURNAL ARTICLES AND INDIVIDUAL CHAPTERS

Abruzzi, Lyn. "What Nursing Has Meant to Me." *La Leche League News* 14 (January–February 1972): 5.

Adago, Catherine. "A Vigil of Hope." *New Beginnings* 8 (March–April 1991): 39.

Aloià, J. F. "Nutritional Reviews: Parathyroid Hormone, 1-25-Dehydroxy, Vitamin D3 and Calcitonin in Women Breastfeeding Twins." *Nature* 43 (October 1985): n.p.

———. "Risk Factors for Postmenopausal Osteoporosis." *American Journal of Medicine* 78 (1985): 95–100.

Andrews, Florence Kellner. "Controlling Motherhood: Observations on the Culture of the La Leche League." *Canadian Review of Sociology and Anthropology* 28, no. 1 (Spring 1991): 84–98.

Applebaum, R. M. "The Obstetrician's Approach to the Breasts and Breastfeeding." *Journal of Reproductive Medicine* 14 (1975): 98–116.

Bacon, C. J., and J. M. Wylie. "Mothers' Attitudes to Infant Feeding at Newcastle General Hospital in Summer 1975." *British Medical Journal* 1, no. 6005 (February 7, 1976): 308–9.

Becker, Mary. "Maternal Feelings: Myth, Taboo, and Child Custody." *Review of Law and Women's Studies* 1 (1992): 142–67.

Bobman, Anne. "A Romantic Ride." *New Beginnings* 5 (January–February 1989): 20.

Bonaparte, Santa. "An Early Weaning." *La Leche League News* 25 (May–June 1983): 50.

Boostrom, Robert. "Baring the Breast: Love, Defilement and Breast-Feeding." *Perspectives in Biology and Medicine* 3 (Spring 1995): 406–22.

Borresen, Kari. "Mary in Catholic Theology." In *Mary in the Churches*, edited by Hans Kung and Jürgen Moltmann, 48–56. Concilium, vol. 168. New York: Seabury Press, 1983.

Byers, T. "Lactation and Breast Cancer: Evidence for Negative Association in Premenopausal Women." *American Journal of Epidemiology* 121 (May 1985): 664–73.

Cahill, Lisa Sowle. "Marriage: Institution, Relationship, Sacrament." In *One Hundred Years of Catholic Social Thought*, edited by John A. Coleman, 103–19. Maryknoll, N.Y.: Orbis, 1991.

Cahill, Mary Ann. "A Backward Glance and a Forward Look." *La Leche League News* 1 (July–August 1958): 1–3.

———. "Mother-Baby Separation." *Leaven* 15 (May–June 1979): 17.

Campion, Donald. "The Church Today." Introduction to *Gaudium et Spes*. In *The Documents of Vatican II*, edited by Walter M. Abbott, 183–98. New York: Guild Press, 1966.

Carson, Mary B. "About Bonding." *La Leche League News* 19 (September–October 1977): 89.

Casebeer, J. B. "Who Shall Treat the Children?" *Archives of Pediatrics* 1 (1884): 735–43.

Chodorow, Nancy, and Susan Cantratto. "The Fantasy of the Perfect Mother." *Social Problems* 23, no. 2 (1976): 54–75.

Chopp, Rebecca. "Feminist Theology." In *A New Handbook of Christian Theology*, edited by Donald W. Musser and Joseph L. Price, 185–91. Nashville: Abingdon Press, 1992.

Christ, Carol. "Margaret Atwood: The Surfacing of Women's Spiritual Quest and Vision." *Signs* 2 (Winter 1976): 316–39.

Coleman, John A. "A Tradition Celebrated, Reevaluated, and Applied." In *One Hundred Years of Catholic Social Thought*, edited by John A. Coleman, 1–10. Maryknoll, N.Y.: Orbis, 1991.

Constantino, Flor. "The Essence of La Leche League." *Leaven* 21 (July–August 1985): 67–68.

"Conversation with Valerie Saiving, A." *Journal of Feminist Studies in Religion* 4 (Fall 1988): 99–108.

Cortes, Ernie. "Reflections on the Catholic Tradition of Family Rights." In *One Hundred Years of Catholic Social Thought*, edited by John A. Coleman, 155–73. Maryknoll, N.Y.: Orbis, 1991.

Countryman, Betty Ann. "New Professional Liaison Department." *Leaven* (September–October 1974): 27.

Crase, Betty. "Making Your Wishes Come True." *New Beginnings* 4 (May–June 1988): 82.

Demestrakopoulas, Stephanie. "The Nursing Mother and Feminine Metaphysics." *Soundings* (Winter 1982): 430–53.

Duffy, John. "Women in the War Industry." *Ave Maria* 56 (July 25, 1942): 99.

"Editorial: Breast-Fed and Bottle-Fed Babies." *Journal of the American Medical Association* 96 (1931): 1231–32.

Eley, R. Cannon. "Medical Progress: Artificial Feeding of Infants." *New England Journal of Medicine* 225 (1941): 230–32.

Elizondo, Virgil. "Mary and the Poor." In *Mary in the Churches*, edited by Hans Kung and Jürgen Moltmann, 59–65. Concilium, vol. 168. New York: Seabury Press, 1983.

E. M. B. "Mothers and Nursing Don't Always Mix." *Chicago Tribune*, August 21, 1959.

Eskuchen, Terry. "Parenting Styles." *New Beginnings* 6 (March–April 1990): 42.

Everman, Jan. "Making a Choice." *New Beginnings* 4 (November–December 1988): 177–78.

Fahey, Rosemary. "Benefits of Being a Leader." *Leaven* (Spring–Summer 1967): 26.

Freed, Gary L. "Time to Teach What We Preach." *Journal of the American Medical Association* 270 (January 13, 1993): 243–44.

Friesen, Delores. "The Welcoming of Jonathan." *La Leche League News* 17 (March–April 1975): 17–18.

Frisbie, Richard. "La Leche League." *Grail* 40 (April 1957): 21–25.

"From the Editor." *Northwest Notes* 4 (March 1969): 2.

Good, Judy, and Susan Phillips. "How Leaders Help Mothers Who Plan Regular Separation from Their Babies." *Leaven* 16 (July–August 1980): 25–26.

Gotsch, Gwen. "Can Breastfeeding Become the Cultural Norm?" *New Beginnings* 4 (November–December 1988): 163–68.

———. "Daddies Are for Fun." *New Beginnings* 8 (July–August 1991): 115.

Gough, Kathleen. "The Origins of the Family." *Journal of Marriage and the Family* (November 1971): 760–68.

Greenley, T. B. "The Management of Infants under a Year Old, Hygienic, Dietetic and Medicinal." *Journal of the American Medical Association* 13 (October 12, 1889): 509–11.

Grobman, Joann Sills. [Untitled]. *La Leche League News* 19 (September–October 1977): 89.

Hahn, Nance L. "Mothering: A Career Perspective." *Leaven* 15 (July–August 1979): 27.

Halkes, Catharina. "Mary and Women." In *Mary in the Churches*, edited by Hans Kung and Jürgen Moltmann, 66–73. Councilium, vol. 168. New York: Seabury Press, 1983.

Harris, Betsy. "Physicians and Leader . . . Working Together." *Leader's Link* (March–April 1979): n.p.

Ing, Roy Ho, and Nicholas Petrakis. "Unilateral Breastfeeding and Cancer." *Lancet* 16 (July 1977): 124–27.

Janssens, Louis. "Norms and Priorities in a Love Ethic." *Louvain Studies* 6 (Spring 1977): 207–38.

Jelliffe, D. B. "Community and Sociopolitical Considerations of Breastfeeding." In *Breast-Feeding and the Mother: Symposium on Breast-Feeding*, 231–55. The Hague: Mouton, 1976.

Johansson, Sheila. "Centuries of Childhood / Centuries of Parenting." *Journal of Family History* 12 (1987): 343–65.

———. "The Moral Imperatives of Christian Marriage." In *One Hundred Years of Catholic Social Thought*, edited by John A. Coleman, 135–54. Maryknoll, N.Y.: Orbis, 1991.

Kassel, Maria. "Mary and the Human Psyche Considered in the Light of Depth Psychology." In *Mary in the Churches*, edited by Hans Kung and Jürgen Moltmann, 74–83. Concilium, vol. 168. New York: Seabury Press, 1983.

Kitzinger, S. "'When Im Seem Bellyful Im Burps and Stops': Breastfeeding Contrasts." *Health Visit* 49 (1976): 34–46.

Kuttner, Robert L. "Worker Rights and Responsibilities in a Changed Competitive Context." In *One Hundred Years of Catholic Social Thought*, edited by John A. Coleman, 234–39. Maryknoll, N.Y.: Orbis, 1991.

"La Leche League Goes to Prison." *Leaven* 18 (November–December 1982): 55–56.

La Leche League International. "Helping Mothers and Babies Everywhere." *Leaven* 18 (January–February 1982): 1–2.

———. "A Special Letter to League Mothers." *Spice Shelf* (Summer 1976): 1–2.

La Leche League of Illinois. "Working with a Leader Applicant." *Spice Shelf* (Fall 1969): 3–4.

La Leche League of Maryland and Virginia. [Untitled]. *Maryland and Virginia News* (1969): n.p.

La Leche League of Ohio. "Some Reminders." *Communiqué* (November 1967): 4.

Ladas, Alice K. "How to Help Mothers Breastfeed." *Clinical Pediatrics* 9 (December 1970): 702–5.

Lamb, M. E., A. M. Frodi, C. P. Hwang, and M. Frodi. "Varying Degrees of Paternal Involvement in Infant Care: Attitudinal and Behavioral Correlates." In *Nontraditional Families: Parenting and Child Development*, edited by M. E. Lamb, 117–38. Hillsdale, N.J.: Erlbaum, 1982.

Leroux, Charles, and Cindy Schreuder. "Handle with Care." *Chicago Tribune*, October 30, 1994, sec. 1, p. 9.

Lewis, Betty. "Managerial Nursing." *New Beginnings* 5 (March–April 1989): 40.

Locklin, Maryanne. "Passionate Advocacy: A Look Back, a Look Forward." *Journal of Human Lactation* 9 (September 1993): 181.

Loomer, Bernard. "Two Conceptions of Power." *Criterion* (Winter 1976): 12–29.

Lorber, J., R. L. Coser, A. S. Rossi, and N. Chodorow. "On *The Reproduction of Mothering*: A Methodological Debate." *Signs* 7, no. 1 (Spring 1981): 482–514.

Loue, Mary. [Untitled]. *Leaven* (Fall–Winter 1966): 28.

Maguire, Daniel C. "The Feminization of God and Ethics." *The Annual* (1982): 1–24.

Mananzan, Mary John. "Education to Femininity or Feminism?" In *The Special Nature of Women*, edited by Anne Carr and Elisabeth Schussler Fiorenza, 28–38. Concilium, vol. 6. Philadelphia: Trinity Press International, 1991.

Matson, Virginia, and Helen Kreigh. "They Wanted to Nurse Their Babies." (This article is preserved without reference to publication or date in the La Leche League Archives.)

Mayer, Linda. "A Loving Partner." *New Beginnings* 4 (November–December 1988): 177.

Mayo, Marilyn. "Breast or Bottle?" *Expecting* (Winter 1993–94): 38–40.

Meara, Hannah. "A Key to Successful Breast-Feeding in a Non-Supportive Culture." *Journal of Nurse-Midwifery* 21, no. 1 (Spring 1976): 20–26.

Meyer, H. "Breast Feeding in the United States." *Clinical Pediatrics* 7 (December 1968): 708.

Meyer-Wilmes, Hedwig. "Women's Nature and Feminine Identity: Theological Legitimations and Feminist Questions." In *Women, Work and Poverty*, edited by Elisabeth S. Fiorenza and Anne E. Carr, 93–101. Concilium, vol. 194(6). New York: Seabury Press, 1987.

Miller, Amata. "The Centennial Encyclical: *Centesimus Annus.*" In NETWORK, *Shaping a New World*, 9–10. Washington, D.C.: Network, 1991.

———. "On the Side of the Poor: Evolution of a Stance." In NETWORK, *Shaping a New World*, 11–12. Washington, D.C.: Network, 1991.

Nash, John. "The Father in Contemporary Culture and Current Psychological Literature." *Child Development* 36 (January 1965): 261–97.

Navin, Ava Wilhite. "A Remarkable Leader." *New Beginnings* 4 (May–June 1988): 84.

Nevins, Joseph V. "Education to Catholic Marriage." *Ecclesiastical Review* 79 (September 1929): 249.

Newton, Niles. "Psychological Differences between Breast and Bottle Feeding." *American Journal of Clinical Nutrition* 24 (1972): 993–1004.

Plaskow, Judith. "Carol Christ on Margaret Atwood: Some Theological Reflections." *Signs* 2 (Winter 1976): 331–39.

Plummer, Linda. Review of *Oneness and Separateness: From Infant to Individual*, by Louise J. Kaplan. *Leaven* 16 (March–April 1980): 11–12.

Pogash, Carol. "The War between Women." *Chicago Tribune*, October 8, 1989, sec. C, p. 4.

Pope, Stephen J. "The Order of Love and Recent Catholic Ethics: A Constructive Proposal." *Theological Studies* 52 (1991): 255–88. (Pope draws his analysis from the *Summa Theologiae*, translated by Fathers of the English Dominican Province, 3 vols. [New York: Benziger Brothers, 1947].)

Quiqley, Lynette. "Our Play Group." *New Beginnings* 1 (May–June 1985): 72.

Radin, Norma. "Primary Caregiving and Role-Sharing Fathers." In *Nontraditional Families: Parenting and Child Development*, edited by M. E. Lamb, 173–204. Hillsdale, N.J.: Erlbaum, 1982.

Richardson, Frank Howard. "How to Nurse Your Baby." *Hygeia* (June 1941): 468–70.

Rivers, Sheryl. "A New School of Thought." *Chicago Tribune*, January 3, 1994, sec. 5, p. 1.

Romano, Randee. "Oxytocin: The Hormone of Love." *New Beginnings* 6 (May–June 1990): 78–79.

Rookey, Hallie S. "All-Natural Ice Milk." *New Beginnings* 6 (September–October 1990): 149.

Rotch, T. M. "The General Principles Underlying All Good Methods of Infant Feeding." *Boston Medical and Surgical Journal* 129 (September 1893): 505–6.

Ruether, Rosemary Radford. "Feminism, Church and Family in the 1980s." *New Blackfriars* 65 (May 1984): 202–12.

———. "An Unrealized Revolution: Searching Scripture for a Model of the Family." *Christianity and Crisis* 43 (1983): 339–404.

Russell, Graeme. "Shared-Caregiving Families: An Australian Study." In *Nontraditional Families: Parenting and Child Development*, edited by M. E. Lamb, 139–71. Hillsdale, N.J.: Erlbaum, 1982.

Sagi, Abraham. "Antecedents and Consequences of Various Degrees of Paternal Involvement in Child Rearing: The Israeli Project." In *Nontraditional Families: Parenting and Child Development*, edited by M. E. Lamb, 205–32. Hillsdale, N.J.: Erlbaum, 1982.

Scheff, Helene. "What Is Development?" *New Beginnings* 6 (September–October 1990): 146.

Schuyler, Joseph B. "Women at Work." *Catholic World* 157 (April 1943): 27–30.

Snitow, Ann. "Feminism and Motherhood: An American Reading." *Feminist Review* 40 (Spring 1992): 32–51.

Spradin, Rebecca. "One and One and Three." *La Leche League News* 19 (May–June 1977): 53.

Stackhouse, Max. "Introduction: Foundations and Purposes." In *On Moral Business*, edited by Dennis McCann, Shirley Roels, and Max Stackhouse. Grand Rapids, Mich.: W. B. Eerdmans, 1995.

Stanton, Nancy. Review of *Who Cares for the Baby?*, by Beatrice Marden Glickman and Nesha Bass Springer. *Leaven* (November–December 1978): 36.

Stewart, David. "A Father Is Born." *La Leche League News* 19 (May–June 1977): 42.

Sweeny, Marlene. "Thirty-five Years Strong: The Same and Changing." *New Beginnings* (January–February 1990): 3–6.

Taylor, Jeremy. "The Duty of Nursing Children." In *The Whole Works of the Right Rev. Jeremy Taylor*, 2:72–81. London: Heber-Eden Editions, 1856. Reprinted in *Child and Family* 8 (Fall 1969): 19–29.

Thomas, J. L. "Catholic Families in a Complex Society: A Cultural Subsystem." *Social Order* 5 (February 1955): 69–82.

———. "Catholic Family in a Complex Society: How to Keep It a Growing Concern." *Social Order* 5 (April 1955): 160–72.

Tompson, Marian. "Note to the Reader." *La Leche League News* 1 (July–August 1958): 2.

Townsend, Sara. "Breastfeeding Gains Popularity in Honduras." *Network* (October 1992): 15–17.

Varencov, Helenka. "The Nursing Madonna: A Cultural Motif." *Child and Family* 8 (Fall 1969): 8–17.

Voyles, Twyalia. "Time to Wean?" *La Leche League News* 25 (March–April 1983): 28.

White, Patti. "The Full Circle." *New Beginnings* 8 (July–August 1991): 110.

Wilber, Charles K. "Incentives and the Organization of Work: Moral Hazards and Trust." In *One Hundred Years of Catholic Social Thought*, edited by John A. Coleman, 212–23. Maryknoll, N.Y.: Orbis, 1991.

Wilson, Linda. "Musings." *La Leche League News* (January–February 1972): 5.

Wood, E. A. "Address on Dietetics." *Journal of the American Medical Association* 11 (July 14, 1888): 37–39.

Work, J. A. "Some of the Causes of the Great Mortality in Infancy and Childhood." *Journal of the American Medical Association* 14 (October 12, 1895): 618–19.

Zappone, Katherine. "Woman's Special Nature: A Different Horizon for Theological Anthropology." In *The Special Nature of Women*, edited by Anne Carr and Elisabeth Schussler Fiorenza, 87–97. Concilium, vol. 6. Philadelphia: Trinity Press International, 1991.

LA LECHE LEAGUE PAMPHLETS AND INSTRUCTIONAL MATERIALS

La Leche League International. *Becoming a La Leche League Leader*. Franklin Park, Ill.: La Leche League International, 1978.

———. *Breastfeeding Peer Counselor Program*. Franklin Park, Ill.: La Leche League International, 1991.

———. "Evaluation Form." In *Application Packet*. Franklin Park, Ill.: La Leche League International, June 1978.

———. *Leader's Handbook*. Franklin Park, Ill.: La Leche League International, 1972.

———. "Letter to Leader." In *Application Packet*. Franklin Park, Ill.: La Leche League International, June 1978.

———. *Statement of Policy* (no. 2). Franklin Park, Ill.: La Leche League International, revised December 1973.

———. *Why Nurse Your Baby?* Franklin Park, Ill.: La Leche League International, n.d.

UNPUBLISHED MATERIALS

Black, Linda S. "The Medicalization of Breastfeeding and Other Intrusions into Motherhood." Paper presented at the La Leche League Fourteenth International Conference, Chicago, July 10–13, 1995.

Cahill, Lisa Sowle. "Sex, Gender and the Family: Challenges for Roman Catholicism." Paper presented at the Religion, Culture, and the Family Project, Chicago, December 6–8, 1991.

Cahill, Mary Ann (founding mother). Interview by author, Franklin Park, Ill., March 3, 1993. Tape recording.

Fazal, Anwar. "The Rebirth of Breastfeeding Worldwide." Paper presented at the La Leche League Fourteenth International Conference, Chicago, July 10–13, 1995.

Froehlich, Edwina (founding mother). Interview by author, Franklin Park, Ill., March 4, 1993. Tape recording.

———. "Nurturing the World through Nurturing Our Families." Paper presented at the La Leche League Fourteenth International Conference, Chicago, July 10–13, 1995.

Gartner, Lawrence. "Two Thousand Years of Medical Advice on Breast Feeding." Paper presented at the annual meeting of the Society of Medical History of Chicago, Chicago, April 13, 1993.

King, Barbara. Letter to the author, March 25, 1980.

Kerwin, Mary Ann (founding mother). Telephone interview by author, March 27, 1993.

Lennon, Viola (founding mother). Interview by author, Franklin Park, Ill., March 4, 1993. Tape recording.

Lopez, Ingrid Carol, Maryanne Stone-Jimenez, Edith Nova Bustos, and Priscilla Stothers. "The Establishment of Mother-to-Mother Support in Economically Disadvantaged and Low-Literate Communities in Developing Areas of the World, Part C, Working and Breastfeeding, Mother-to-Mother Support and the Health Care Community." Paper presented at the La Leche League Fourteenth International Conference, Chicago, July 10–13, 1995.

Newman, Jack. "Mutual Respect in the Health Care Community: Lay and Professional Care Providers Working Together to Support the Breastfeeding Family." Paper presented at the La Leche League Fourteenth International Conference, Chicago, July 10–13, 1995.

Schuck, Michael Joseph. "The Content and Coherence of Roman Catholic Encyclical Social Teaching, 1740–1987." Ph.D. dissertation, University of Chicago, 1988.

Thevenin, Tine. "Mothering and Fathering: The Gender Difference in Childrearing."

Paper presented at the La Leche League Fourteenth International Conference, Chicago, July 10–13, 1995.

Tompson, Marian (founding mother). Interview by author, Evanston, Ill., March 25, 1993.

Wagner, Betty (founding mother). Interview by author, Franklin Park, Ill., March 3, 1993.

Ward, Jule. Letter to Barbara King, n.d.

White, Mary (founding mother). Interview by author, River Forest, Ill., March 24, 1993.

index

· ·